The Nurse's Guide to Teaching Diabetes Self-Management

Rita G. Mertig, MS, RNC, CNS, is a professor of nursing at John Tyler Community College in Chester, Virginia. She teaches Maternal-Newborn Nursing in the third semester which includes maternity nursing, nursing of children and psychiatric/mental health nursing. She also teaches nutrition and test-taking in nursing. She has taught diabetes in the beginning medical-surgical nursing course and fluid and electrolytes in the fundamentals of nursing course, as well as a health assessment course. Her prior teaching experience includes baccalaureate, diploma, and practical nursing programs.

She graduated from Georgetown University with a Bachelor of Science in nursing degree and received her Master of Science degree from the University of California, San Francisco Medical Center School of Nursing. She is a clinical nurse specialist and is certified in maternity-newborn nursing. She also is a certified childbirth educator and is a member of the American Association of Diabetes Educators, the Association of Women's Health, Obstetrics and Neonatal Nurses Association, and Sigma Theta Tau. She authored *Teaching Nursing in an Associate Degree Program*, has contributed to chapters in fundamentals of nursing and nursing skills textbooks, and has written the chapter on diabetes in *Nurses Guide to Consumer Health Web Sites*. She has also been a reviewer for fundamentals of nursing, nursing skills, and maternity nursing textbooks as well as a test bank book.

The Nurse's Guide to Teaching Diabetes Self-Management

Rita Girouard Mertig, MS, RNC, CNS

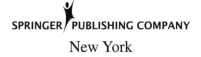

SPRINGER PUBLISHING COMPANY
New York

Springer Publishing Company, LLC
11 West 42nd Street
New York, NY 10036

Acquisitions Editor: Sheri W. Sussman

Managing Editor: Mary Ann McLaughlin

Project Manager: Carol Cain

Cover design by Joanne E. Honigman

Typeset by Apex Publishing, LLC

07   08   09   10/   5   4   3   2

Library of Congress Cataloging-in-Publication Data

Mertig, Rita G.
  The nurse's guide to teaching diabetes self-management
    p. ; cm.
  Includes bibliographical references and index.
  ISBN 0-8261-0225-5
  1. Diabetes—Nursing. 2. Patient education. 3. Self-care, Health. I. Title.
  [DNLM: 1. Diabetes Mellitus—therapy—Nurses' Instruction. 2. Diabetes Mellitus—psychology—Nurses' Instruction. 3. Nurse-Patient Relations—Nurses' Instruction. 4. Patient Education—Nurses' Instruction. 5. Self Care—psychology—Nurses' Instruction. WK 815 M575n 2006]
  RC660.M47 2006
  616.4'620231—dc22

                                                    2006018589

Printed in the United States of America by Bang Printing

Contents

List of Figures   *ix*

List of Tables   *x*

Preface   *xi*

Acknowledgments   *xiii*

Introduction   *xiv*

Part I The Diabetes Conundrum   1

1. Diabetes: The Basics   3
   How Insulin Works   3
   Classification of Diabetes   5
   Diagnostic Criteria   8

2. Treatment: Medical Nutrition Therapy   11
   Nutrition   11
   Weight Loss   14
   Old Food Pyramid Versus 2005 Dietary Guidelines   15
   Carb Counting   16
   Alcohol: Pros and Cons   17
   Sick-Day Management   18

3. Treatment: Physical Activity   21
   Benefits of Exercise   21
   Potential Problems With Exercise   23

4. Treatment: Medication   27
   Oral Antidiabetic Medications   28
   Injectable Antidiabetic Medication   34
   Inhaled Insulin   46

5. Glycemic Control 51
Hyperglycemia 53
Hypoglycemia 56
Blood Glucose Monitoring 59

6. The Cure Is Near 65
Research in the Prevention and Cure of Type 1 Diabetes 65
Research in the Prevention and Cure of Type 2 Diabetes 71
How a New Drug or Product Gets Approved 71

Part II Diabetes Self-Management 77

7. The Nurse as Teacher 79
What Do Clients With Diabetes Need To Know? 80
Assessment Guidelines 82
Goals of Client Education 82
Nursing Interventions Using Learning Principles 85
Evaluating Teaching 93

8. Children With Diabetes and Their Parents 97
Kearsten Mauney, BA, MT
What Is it Like to Have a Child With Diabetes? 97
Ages and Stages 99

9. Adolescents With Diabetes 107
Beverly Baliko, PhD, RN
Balancing Parental Involvement 108
Nonadherence in Adolescents With Diabetes 109

10. Diabetes in Adults With Special Needs 115
Diabetes and Pregnancy 115
Diabetes in the Elderly 123

11. Diabetes and Mental Illness 129
Beverly Baliko, PhD, RN
Diabetes and Depression 130
Diabetes and Chronic, Severe Mental Illnesses 135
Teaching and Motivating Clients With Mental Illnesses 138

12. Client Noncompliance 143
Definitions 143
Financial Considerations 144

Physical Limitations   145
Deficient Knowledge   145
Literacy   146
Culture   147
Religious Constraints   149
Support System   149
Denial   150
Anger   152
Depression   153
Fatalism   153
Self-Determination   154

Index   159

Beverly Baliko, PhD, RN, has worked with adults and adolescents with psychiatric-mental health issues for 15 years. She has been a nurse educator for 5 years, teaching in nursing in associate degree, diploma, and baccalaureate programs. She received her bachelor's and master's degree at the Medical University of South Carolina and obtained her PhD in Nursing at Virginia Commonwealth University. She is currently an assistant professor at the University of South Carolina.

Kearsten H. Mauney, BA, MT, is a teacher in Henrico County Public Schools and has 13 years' experience in education. She teaches 6th grade Mathematics at Wilder Middle School. She has also taught Language Arts and Social Studies at the middle school level. She graduated with a Bachelor of Arts in Music Performance from Mary Washington College and received her Master of Teaching degree from Virginia Commonwealth University.

She is a mother to nine-year-old twin boys, Patrick and Brennan. Her son, Brennan, was diagnosed with Type I diabetes at the age of 2. At the age of 7, Brennan was found to have a learning disability. Her experience as a teacher and as a parent of a child diagnosed with diabetes at a young age provides a unique perspective into the thoughts, concerns, and fears of parents whose children have been diagnosed with diabetes.

Kearsten is also a member of the Tuckahoe Jaycees in Virginia. She is a national winner for the United States Junior Chamber of Commerce in the areas of public speaking and writing. Her award-winning speech prompted fundraising efforts for JDRF within her local chapter. She has served as Competitions Program Manager for the Virginia Jaycees, and she is currently their Annual Achievement Awards Program Manager.

List of Figures

1.1   How the Pancreas Regulates Blood Sugar   4
2.1   Body Mass Index   15
7.1   Diabetes Questionnaire   86
7.2   Diabetes Mellitus Client Questionnaire   90

List of Tables

1.1	Diabetes Classifications	5
3.1	Diabetic Complications and Exercise	25
4.1	Oral Antidiabetic Medication	29
4.2	Types of Insulin	38
4.3	Conversion Table for Doses of Symlin (Pramlintide) for Subcutaneous Injection	45
5.1	Correlation Between A1C Level and Mean Plasma Glucose Levels on Multiple Testing Over 2–3 Months	52
5.2	Factors That Affect Blood Sugar	55
5.3	Rules to Follow for Glycemic Control	60
6.1	Four Phases of Investigational Drug Studies	73
7.1	Major Components of Diabetes Self-Management Education	81
7.2	Learning Principles for the Adult Learner	89
8.1	Signs and Symptoms of Hypoglycemia and Hyperglycemia in Children	101
8.2	What Should Be Included in a DMMP	103
10.1	Diagnostic Criteria for Gestational Diabetes	120

Preface

Nurses are charged with the responsibility to teach newly diagnosed clients with diabetes and to review with others the multiple aspects of diabetes care. Diabetes management has changed greatly in the last few years with regard to diet, medication, and exercise recommendations. It is difficult for nurses to keep up and to help clients work with the new research that is improving the lives of diabetics and decreasing or postponing the many long-term complications. Too many nurses do not practice teaching and learning strategies as applied to the child, parent, and adult learner. Most are frustrated by the apparent lack of compliance of some clients with diabetes and fail to understand motivation theory and the need to individualize their teaching.

As a person with diabetes and a professor of nursing, my purpose in writing this book is to help nurses learn about new strategies to better manage diabetes, as well as to guide them in the practice of individualizing their approach to clients using theories of learning and motivation. Nurses have more access to clients than any other healthcare professional and are generally more approachable. The diabetic teaching they render may make all the difference for their clients' future healthcare. The impact that well-informed nurses can have on diabetic self-management is incalculable. This book was also written to inspire and empower all who deal with diabetes daily on a personal level.

When I started researching the material for this book, I realized that my title needed to change from "What Nurses Need to Know About Diabetes" to the present title. Nurses need to stay as current as possible on the topic of diabetes because many of the clients they care for have diabetes. No matter where nurses work, diabetes is either their clients' primary management concern or it complicates any other physical or mental difficulties for which they are being treated. Part 1 of this book deals with the current ins and outs of diabetes management. This is the science of diabetes care that nurses must know. However, nursing is not just about understanding a disease entity. Nursing is also an art. The art of nursing comes with experience and practice. It comes from an in-depth understanding of people and how to relate to them as individuals.

Part 2 of this book deals with the application of teaching and learning principles to individuals dealing with diabetes throughout the life span. One size does not fit all, and so-called canned teaching sessions without assessing the individual needs of each client will fail in most cases. Nurses *teach* every time they walk into a client's room. Your "patient" and his or her family watch you and listen to your every word. What is it that they are getting out of their experience with you? If you ask good questions, adapt your care accordingly, and teach to meet their stated needs, they perceive that you really care. The clients and their families are more likely to be empowered to learn about this condition and its treatment and work at self-management. If you treat them like any other "patient" with diabetes, they may well be turned off by your perceived indifference and either go it alone or become noncompliant. Nurses have more power to effect change than we can possibly imagine. It is my hope that Part 2 will awaken or encourage the ideals that lead you to nursing school in the first place. True, there is a long-standing nursing shortage. However, the long hours and overwork cannot beat these ideals out of you unless you allow them to. Let the chapters in Part 2 of this book help you to develop new strategies for really making a difference in people's lives.

For fellow diabetics who read this book, I hope you learn what you need to know from the current information about diabetes in Part 1. More importantly, I want the chapters in Part 2 that apply to you to inspire you to ask more questions and demand more individualized care from nurses wherever you interact with them. You need to expect and demand the respect you deserve and the answers you need to "be the best that you can be." If nothing else, you can show them this book and encourage them to read it. "It takes a village" to learn and deal with your life with diabetes. If others in health care, who should be helping you on your road to better health, are not helping you, complain. Make your needs known even if they do not ask about them. Make it personal, because it really *is* in the end.

Rita G. Mertig

Acknowledgments

I would like to thank in a formal way the following people who made it possible to write this book:

Dr. Ursula Springer, who gave me the opportunity to write this second book, and Sally Barhydt, my contact person at Springer Publishing, who was so generous with her time, advice, and encouragement.

My family, who gave of their time generously and were always willing to rearrange planned family events to suit my writing schedule; I owe them my sanity. My adult daughters, Karen and Kelley, generously gave me the benefit of their wisdom in editing several chapters. Kelley, a budding author herself, has spent many hours and days editing large portions of this manuscript and advising me on my computer concerns and on the consistency of the book. My husband, Bob, took over all the cooking, cleaning, and grocery shopping chores, despite his new job, so I could pursue my goal of completing this manuscript.

My boss, Deborah Ulmer, who understood my passion to write this book and refrained from asking me to do more than what was expected of a faculty member. She made this last year of teaching and writing doable.

Dr. Solomon Klioze, PhD, director, cardiovascular and metabolic diseases, clinical research and development at Pfizer Global Pharmaceuticals, who so patiently helped me to understand the research into inhaled insulin and to write about it.

Bev Baliko and Kearsten Mauney, who consented to write chapters that I did not have the expertise to write; I am very grateful. My friend and typist, Donna Davis, who put up with my handwriting and my many arrows and odd directions; thanks for saving me a lot of time and energy. Thanks also to Patsy Bragg, who generously acted as courier.

Lastly, I'd like to thank the members of the Richmond Area Pump Club and the many people struggling with diabetes with whom I have spoken. They shared their stories, hopes, and difficulties and helped me to put into words what they want nurses to know.

Rita G. Mertig

Introduction

When life hands you a lemon, you make lemonade.
When I was in nursing school learning about diabetes mellitus and all of its complications, I decided that if I had diabetes I would never have children. I thought it was a horrible legacy to pass on to future generations. When I was diagnosed with diabetes in my late 30s, I already had children, and the guilt I experienced was enormous. I also went through all of Dr. Elisabeth Kübler-Ross's "stages of grief" (denial, anger, bargaining, depression, and acceptance). They are as pertinent to loss of perceived health as they are to loss of a body part or of life itself when a terminal diagnosis is given. The plans I had made for my life, my family, and my career would never be realized. Not me! I wasted 3 months of my life in denial, eating very few carbohydrates, exercising after every meal, and seeing another physician for an alternative diagnosis, all to no avail. I was also angry at everyone I knew who smoked, was overweight, or who did not exercise, and I was very angry with God. Why me? I took care of my body and look at the thanks I got.

When I finally decided that "yes, it is me, but ... ," the bargaining began. OK, as long as I don't have to take insulin, I can manage life with diabetes. Meanwhile, I was reading everything I could get my hands on and asking my physician a million questions. This was back in the days before widespread use of glucose monitors. Human insulin had just come on the market, and the only oral hypoglycemic drugs were first-generation sulfonylureas such as Orinase, Tolinase, and Diabinase, drugs that are rarely used today. When two tablets of Diabinase, a maximum dose, failed to decrease my blood sugar, I was put on insulin. I gave myself my first shot of insulin in the examination room under the supervision of a nurse. I did it perfectly, having given many injections to others during my nursing career. I had also taught and supervised many student nurses giving injections for several years. However, after this first injection, I cried for 20 to 30 minutes. It didn't hurt, but my denial was over. I could no longer pretend my diabetes pills were vitamins. My bargaining had failed. I did have diabetes and would be giving myself insulin injections for the rest of my probably shortened life. It might also mean I'd be on dialysis, perhaps blind and missing a few toes, or worse, before I finally died. To put it mildly, I was very depressed.

I don't know what helped me to turn my attitude around, to finally accept my fate and work at making the best of what I considered to be a dismal future. Maybe it was the hope I received from all of my research about diabetes management. Maybe it was my husband's faith in my ability to overcome adversity. He actually told me that not only would I conquer this, but I would probably profit from it. In actuality, I have spoken about diabetes to hundreds of student nurses, nurses, and persons with diabetes, and have now written this book. Another factor that helped me to come to grips with this diagnosis was that I had to be a positive role model for my children just in case I had passed on this hereditary disease. I had to demonstrate that there was "life after diagnosis."

I have detailed my coming to terms with this disease to help healthcare professionals who read this book to understand how the grieving process applies to a diagnosis of a chronic illness like diabetes, the emotional and physical impact of such a turn of events, and the enormous energy it takes to achieve acceptance so as to work toward the best possible outcome. Please remember my story when you read chapter 12 on client noncompliance.

To those readers who share my diagnosis, I hope you recognize some of your own struggles in my tale and know that you are not alone. The more you share your own feeling and fears, the faster you will move toward acceptance and the better you will be able to work toward achieving the most positive state of wellness possible.

I have been attempting to write this book for years. My first draft started out as a chronological account of my life with diabetes. Such chapters as "Life After Diagnosis" and "Six Months and Counting" helped me to deal with what I was experiencing and how I was evolving as a person. This was more of a journal than the book that you now have in your hands. Several years ago, as I was becoming an "expert" on the subject, I started to write about the new research in diabetes management: new medication and insulins, new dietary guidelines and therapies on the horizons. I gave these handouts to my students so that they could be aware of and look forward to the implementation of cutting-edge technology for diabetes management. Each year I added more and more to the list as research on diabetes escalated. My original two-page handout grew to ten pages, even though I moved some of the items into my lecture because they were now standards of care. That project alone was very empowering to me and to my students who were in the process of becoming tomorrow's nurses. As I shared this handout with those who attended my support group for diabetics, I hoped they, too, were encouraged by the giant leaps forward in the management of their condition.

Part I

The Diabetes Conundrum

What is in a name? Well, as it turns out, quite a bit. The American Diabetes Association has been reclassifying and renaming the types of diabetes over the years as more is understood about the pathology and etiology of each. A major effort was made in 1997 to get rid of old and misleading nomenclature. *Type 1 diabetes* is no longer called *juvenile onset diabetes* because people like me are being diagnosed in their 40s and older. Likewise, *type 2 diabetes* is not thought of as just *adult onset diabetes* because obese children as young as 4 years old meet the criteria. Also treatment with insulin is not the deciding factor between type 1 and type 2 diabetes because insulin is but one of the many medications appropriately used to treat persons with type 2 diabetes. And what in the world is all of this talk about prediabetes? There might even be a type 1.5 diabetes. Expect to read more about both in the coming months and years.

What we all must focus on is the very distinct pathology differentiating the two main forms of diabetes. We must continually remain as updated and current as possible. Why is this important? Knowing what kind of diabetes a person has will help a nurse to anticipate problems, use strategies to prevent these complications, troubleshoot to decide what is going on, and apply correct interventions. For instance, a person with type 1 diabetes is more prone to rapid changes in blood sugar than someone with type 2 diabetes. A client with type 2 who is taking insulin or an oral medication that increases production of insulin is more prone to low blood sugar than someone who is controlled by diet and exercise or by an oral agent that increases tissue sensitivity to the insulin.

Chapters 1 though 5 of this book explore the ins and outs of diabetes so that nurses and clients will understand, in more depth, what is currently known about this mystifying disease. Before nurses can teach clients how to live with diabetes, they must first understand the ramifications of each type of diabetes diagnosed.

1

Diabetes: The Basics

Diabetes mellitus is a group of metabolic diseases characterized by hyperglycemia resulting from defects in insulin secretion, insulin action, or both. The chronic hyperglycemia of diabetes is associated with long-term damage, dysfunction, and failure of various organs, especially the eyes, kidneys, nerves, heart, and blood vessels. (American Diabetes Association [ADA], 2006b, p. S43)

In the fall of 2005 the Centers for Disease Control and Prevention (CDC) estimated that 20.8 million people in the United States have *diabetes mellitus*. Of this number, 14.6 million are diagnosed, thus leaving 6.2 million, or 30% of the total, as yet undiagnosed (National Diabetes Information Clearinghouse [NDIC], 2006). Prior to the 1997 changes made in the diagnostic criteria, it was once estimated that half of all persons with diabetes did not know they had the disease. The 1997 American Diabetes Association diagnostic and classification criteria lowered the fasting blood sugar from 140 mg/dl (milligrams per deciliter) to 126 mg/dl, resulting in many more people being diagnosed and treated. The goal was to identify and treat as many persons as possible to prevent long-term complications. It seems that what you do not know can and will hurt you. Nurses should apply this concept to their own lives and impart it to clients who have or are at risk for diabetes.

HOW INSULIN WORKS

Insulin is a protein and a hormone secreted by the beta cells found throughout the pancreas. When blood sugar rises after a meal, insulin is secreted to help glucose (blood sugar) move into the cells of the body to be used as fuel. If there is more glucose than needed for cellular energy, insulin helps sugar to fill storage places in the liver and skeletal muscles for later use. Glucose is stored there as glycogen. When the amount of glucose in the blood exceeds these two needs, the rest is stored in fat cells, causing weight gain. Another role for insulin is to prevent inappropriate release of glycogen from the liver when it is not needed. If blood sugars drop, for example, from prolonged exercise or a skipped meal, another pancreatic hormone, glucagon, is released to allow the stored glycogen to be released from the liver (see Figure 1.1) to maintain normal blood glucose levels. This is very important because the cells of the brain and nervous system only burn glucose for energy. The rest of the body can function by burning fat and protein for energy in the absence of blood glucose, but the brain cannot.

The beta cells that produce insulin and the alpha cells that produce glucagon are part of the islets of Langerhans that are scattered throughout the pancreas. This fact is important to remember as you read in chapter 6 about the new islet cell transplantation being used to reverse type 1 diabetes. Another important fact to remember is that in a normal pancreas, only approximately one-fourth of the beta cells are needed to keep blood sugars within normal range. The other three-fourths may be called upon when more insulin is needed, for example, when blood glucose load is high, when stress and other hormones increase the release of stored glycogen, or when the body is fighting an infection or other physical condition such as an injury or

FIGURE 1.1 HOW THE PANCREAS REGULATES BLOOD SUGAR

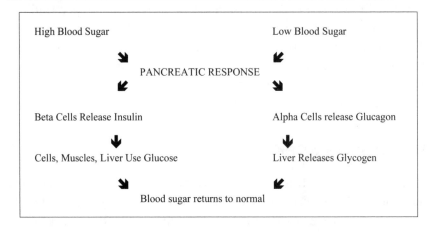

pregnancy. Only when the need for insulin outstrips the supply does blood sugar rise.

CLASSIFICATION OF DIABETES

The pathology that causes each type of diabetes is very different, which should explain why a person with type 2 diabetes cannot change to a type 1 simply because insulin is prescribed to control blood sugar. (See Table 1.1 for differences.)

TABLE 1.1   Diabetes Classifications

	Cause	Fasting blood sugar	Heredity	Insulin production
Normal		70–99 mg/dl		
Prediabetes	Decreased insulin sensitivity	100–125 mg/dl	Very strong	Increased
Type 1	Autoimmune destruction of beta cells	126 mg/dl & up	Not common	Very little
Type 2	Insulin resistance, inadequate amount of insulin	126 mg/dl & up	Very strong	Increased then decreased
Gestational diabetes	Pancreatic hormones cause insulin resistance, insufficient insulin	Abnormal OGTT @ 26–32 weeks	Very strong	Increased
Other (pancreatitis, pancreatic and other cancers, drugs such as prednisone, thiazide diuretics)	Abnormal production of hormones causing insulin resistance	126 mg/dl & up	Sometimes	Decreased

Type 1 diabetes is an autoimmune disease in which the body's own immune system attacks and destroys the beta cells of the pancreas. Thus, in a short span of time from weeks to a few years, the body does not even have the one-fourth of beta cells functioning to prevent a rise in blood sugar. These are not the clients that live for years with undiagnosed diabetes. Clients with type 1 diabetes are diagnosed relatively quickly due to the symptoms of a potentially life-threatening ketoacidosis. When the body ceases to produce sufficient insulin, the cells are starved of their preferred fuel, glucose. The body then begins to burn fat and then protein for energy. The breakdown of fat produces fatty acids and ketones that begin to poison the body. Burning fat and protein reduces fat and lean muscle mass, causing life-threatening weight loss. The body is literally wasting away because the cells have no way of getting to the ever-rising sugar in the blood without insulin to transport it past the cell wall. And as if that was not bad enough, the high blood glucose increases the concentration of the blood so water is pulled from cells and interstitial fluid (fluid around the cells) to dilute the sugar concentration. Kidneys then excrete some of the excess sugar and water as very sweet urine (glycosuria). Without injections of insulin, the body and its cells become very dehydrated, to the point of multiorgan failure. Prior to the discovery of insulin in the 1920s, children with this disease all died. Today, persons with type 1 diabetes account for only 5–10% of those with diabetes, and with proper treatment they can live long, productive lives.

Type 2 diabetes, on the other hand, stems from cellular insulin resistance, an insufficient amount of insulin to overcome this resistance, or a production of insulin that the body cannot use efficiently. For many it is a combination of all three factors. Insulin resistance is often found in persons who are obese. Those obese persons who have not inherited the gene for type 2 diabetes simply produce a large amount of insulin to overcome this resistance and maintain normal blood sugar levels. When type 2 diabetes runs in the family, obesity often results in a diagnosis. According to Christopher Saudek and Simeon Margolis, "About 80% of people with type 2 diabetes are overweight or obese, and the risk of type 2 diabetes rises as a person's weight increases" (Saudek & Margolis, 2006, p. 7). Because this form of diabetes has a strong genetic component, the population at risk for developing type 2 diabetes includes members of the following ethnic groups:

- African Americans
- Asian Americans
- Pacific Islanders such as Hawaiians and Filipinos
- Native Americans (American Indians)
- Mexican Americans

In addition, all overweight and obese individuals have an increased risk of developing metabolic syndrome, formerly called *syndrome X*. The components of this syndrome include obesity, dyslipidemia (low HDLs and high triglycerides), hypertension, and insulin resistance. This syndrome affects at least one out of every five overweight people and increases their risk of being diagnosed with type 2 diabetes (ADA, 2006b, S43–S48).

Gestational diabetes mellitus (GDM) only occurs during pregnancy. It occurs in about 4% of all pregnancies in the United States, resulting in about 135,000 cases diagnosed each year. Ninety percent of all women who have pregnancies complicated by diabetes have gestational diabetes (ADA, n.d.). Women who are overweight or obese, have a family history of type 2 diabetes, and/or are from the high-risk population listed above have a much greater risk of developing gestational diabetes than the general population. Pregnancy and the resulting placental hormones cause some degree of insulin resistance in all women. However, a healthy pancreas is able to produce more and more insulin to keep blood sugars within normal range as the pregnancy advances. Today it is recommended that all but low-risk women be given a 50 gram Glucola, one-hour glucose challenge test as a screening tool between 24 and 28 weeks of gestation because controlling blood glucose during pregnancy enhances maternal and fetal health. Women who have been diagnosed with gestational diabetes have an increased risk for developing type 2 diabetes later in life, often within 5–10 years of pregnancy (ADA, 2006b). Diabetes in pregnancy is covered more thoroughly in chapter 10.

There is a fourth classification of diabetes termed "other," which encompasses those who have a diseased pancreas caused by cancer or infection and those with drug-induced hyperglycemia as is often the case with chronic use of prednisone or other corticosteroids.

In recent years we have heard a lot about *prediabetes*, a term that has replaced *impaired glucose tolerance (IGT)* and *impaired fasting glucose (IFG)* to increase the attention of both health care providers and clients to the fact that time is running out to prevent future diabetes and *cardiovascular disease (CVD)* (Saudek & Margolis, 2006). Prior to developing type 2 diabetes, most clients have had difficulty with glucose tolerance, perhaps for years. This includes a number of people who have metabolic syndrome. Research has shown that organ damage often begins during the prediabetes years. Normal fasting blood sugar once was 70–109 mg/dl, and impaired fasting glucose was 110–125 mg/dl. In 2003, these criteria were lowered to help motivate those with prediabetes to follow guidelines and prevent or delay the diagnosis of type 2 diabetes and long-term complications. These guidelines include weight loss, exercise, and lifestyle modifications. There are about 40 million Americans diagnosed with prediabetes today. As stated in the Johns Hopkins White Papers on diabetes, "Without lifestyle changes or medication, many of them will develop type 2 diabetes in the next 10 years" (Saudek & Margolis, 2006, p. 8). The hope is that, if forewarned, clients will make the changes in their life to lower fasting blood sugar to less than 100 mg/dl and that health care practitioners will be more concerned about the health consequences to their patients in the years prior to their official diagnosis of type 2 diabetes.

DIAGNOSTIC CRITERIA

Most people with diabetes are diagnosed with a fasting blood glucose of 126 mg/dl or higher or a random blood glucose of 200 mg/dl. According to the American Diabetes Association, "FPG [fasting plasma glucose] is the preferred test to diagnose diabetes in children and non-pregnant adults" (ADA, 2006a, p. S6). Common symptoms of diabetes that might initiate a blood glucose test include excessive urination, excessive thirst, weight loss despite cravings for sweets (type 1), fatigue, skin lesions that do not heal, repeat infection, and any end organ damage associated with chronic diabetic complication, particularly cardiovascular and neuropathic problems (type 2). Current American Diabetes Association recommendations for screening people without symptoms include a fasting blood sugar for all individuals 45 years old and older and, if normal, repeating this test every 3 years. Screening should be done earlier than 45 years and/or be done more frequently for those who have any of the following risk factors:

- overweight body mass index (BMI > 25 kg/m^2)
- habitually physically inactive

- first degree relative with diabetes (parent, sibling, child)
- member of a high-risk ethnic population (e.g., African American, Asian American, Pacific Islander, Native American, Mexican American)
- delivered a baby weighing > 9 pounds or diagnosed with gestational diabetes (GDM)
- hypertension (> 140/90 mm Hg)
- HDL cholesterol < 35 mg/dl and/or triglyceride level > 250 mg/dl
- polycystic ovary syndrome (PCOS)
- impaired glucose tolerance (IGT) or impaired fasting glucose (IFG) on previous testing
- any other clinical condition associated with insulin resistance
- history of vascular disease (ADA, 2006b, S43–S48)

Because the incidence of type 2 diabetes in adolescents and children has increased dramatically in the last 10 years, those who meet the criteria listed below are thus at increased risk of developing type 2 diabetes in childhood and should be tested at puberty or age 10, whichever comes first, and retested every 2 years using a fasting blood sugar.

- overweight (BMI > 85th percentile for age and sex, weight for height > 85th percentile, or weight > 120% of ideal for height)

plus any two of the following risk factors:

- family history of type 2 diabetes in first- or second-degree relative
- race/ethnicity (African American Asian American, Pacific Islander, Native American, Mexican American)
- signs of insulin resistance or conditions associated with insulin resistance (acanthosis nigricans, hypertension, dyslipidemia, or polycystic ovary syndrome) (ADA, 2006b, S43–S48)

Children who present with signs and symptoms of diabetes probably have type 1 and are in immediate danger of developing diabetic ketoacidosis.

Because what we do not know about our health can and does cause damage to glucose-sensitive organs, diagnosis of anyone at risk for diabetes and treatment at the earliest possible opportunity are critical.

REFERENCES

American Diabetes Association. (n.d.). *Gestational diabetes.* Retrieved February 18, 2006 from http://www.diabetes.org/gestational-diabetes.jsp

American Diabetes Association. (2006a). Standards of medical care in diabetes—2006. *Diabetes Care, 29,* S4–S42.

American Diabetes Association. (2006b). Diagnosis and classification of diabetes mellitus. *Diabetes Care, 29,* S43–S48.

National Diabetes Information Clearinghouse. (2006). Total prevalence of diabetes in the United States, all ages, 2005. *National diabetes statistics.* Retrieved January 8, 2006, from http://www.diabetes.niddk.nih.gov/dm/pubs/statistics/index.htm

Saudek, C. D., & Margolis, S. (2006). *Johns Hopkins white papers: Diabetes.* Redding, CT: Medletter Associates.

2

Treatment: Medical Nutritional Therapy

Diabetics *have* to do what everyone else *ought* to do.

The goals for treatment for diabetes are to prevent or delay long-term complications while minimizing acute manifestations such as hypoglycemia. Nutrition, exercise, and medication (when needed) are the cornerstones of successfully treating all classifications of diabetes. In addition to diet and physical exercise, lifestyle modifications also include smoking cessation and normalization of blood pressure and blood cholesterol (ADA, 2006). Nurses need to remind their clients that these are goals of a healthy lifestyle for all people, not just those diagnosed with diabetes.

Early on in my career as a diabetic, a very wise physician said to me that which I have quoted above. It changed my life and my attitude toward myself and this disease. As I attempted to control my blood sugars by eating correctly, exercising, and taking multiple injections of insulin, I felt superior to my peers instead of feeling sorry for myself. I then felt I was choosing to live a healthy lifestyle instead of being forced into it. Sometimes bad things can have good consequences.

NUTRITION

Diet is simply what we eat, good, bad, or indifferent. We can have a healthy or unhealthy diet. This word, by itself, has no negative connotations except what we choose to give it. It can be high fat, high carbohydrate, high fast food, high junk food, high calorie, or restrictive in terms of all of the above, or so low in calories as to deprive our body of the nutrients to sustain life. So focusing on nutrition and avoiding the negative images the word diet has come to evoke may improve attitudes and motivation to make healthier food choices.

The American Diabetes Association's Standards of Medical Care in Diabetes—2006 recommends the following lifestyle modifications to prevent or delay the diagnosis of type 2 diabetes:

- Individuals at high risk for developing diabetes need to become aware of the benefits of modest weight loss and participating in regular physical activity.
- Patients with impaired glucose tolerance (IGT) should be given counseling on weight loss as well as instruction for increasing physical activity.
- Patients with impaired fasting glucose (IFG) should be given counseling on weight loss as well as instruction for increasing physical activity.
- Follow-up counseling appears important for success.
- Monitoring for the development of diabetes in those with pre-diabetes should be performed every 1–2 years.
- Close attention should be given to, and appropriate treatment given for, other cardiovascular disease (CVD) risk factors (e.g., tobacco use, hypertension, dyslipidemia). (ADA, 2006, p. S18)

Medical nutritional therapy to achieve and maintain appropriate weight for age, gender, and height must begin with a thorough evaluation of a client's dietary history. It must take into consideration culture, lifestyle, finances, and a person's readiness to learn and change.

Blood sugar is influenced by the amount and type of carbohydrates consumed and whether protein and fat are eaten as part of a meal. For instance, an orange is digested and metabolized more slowly than orange juice and takes longer to increase blood sugar. An orange eaten after cereal and milk or eggs and sausage takes even longer. Protein and fat eaten with carbohydrate foods slow down the absorption of carbohydrate.

"Although dietary carbohydrate is the major contributor to postprandial glucose concentration, it is an important source of energy, water-soluble vitamins and minerals, and fiber. Thus, in agreement with the National Academy of Sciences–Food and Nutrition Board, a recommended range of carbohydrate intake is 45–65% of total calories. In addition, because the brain and central nervous system have an absolute requirement for glucose as an energy source, restricting total carbohydrate to <130 g/day is not recommended" (ADA, 2006, p. S11). These carbohydrates come from fruit (fructose), milk (lactose), starches such as bread, pasta, and starchy vegetables (corn, peas, and all kinds of beans), and table sugar (sucrose). Yes, people with diabetes can eat sugar. The body metabolizes sugar as a carbohydrate. Yet all carbs are not created equally. The empty carbohydrate calories in regular sodas and sugary desserts and snacks contain no nutritive value and should be limited. In addition, desserts and snacks with sugar or high fructose corn syrup also usually have a high fat content, contributing to increased calories and weight gain.

Anyone taking insulin should try to match the number of carbohydrates in a meal or snack with the appropriate amount of insulin (see chapter 4). Fiber is a complex carbohydrate that does not get absorbed in the body so technically should be subtracted from the total. Fiber increases the speed with which food travels through the digestive system, helps to retain bulk and water in the stool as it enters the rectum, and stimulates the urge to defecate, thus preventing constipation.

Fats are a very important part of our diet. They help the absorption of fat-soluble vitamins and provide essential fatty acids (fatty acids the body needs but cannot manufacture). They provide concentrated stored energy and fuel muscle movement. Fat cells pad internal organs and insulate the body against temperature extremes. They also form the major component of cell membranes and are the raw material from which hormones, enzymes, bile, and vitamin D are made. Fats also stimulate appetite, make meats tender, and contribute to satiety. The problem is that they provide 9 calories per gram and contribute to weight gain more than any other nutrient. The American Heart Association, the American Cancer Society, and the American Diabetes Association (2006) recommend that fat should be limited to 25–35% of calories per day and < 7% should be from saturated fat of animal products such as meat, poultry, and full-fat dairy products. Trans fatty acids in any oils that are hydrogenated or partially hydrogenated should be avoided altogether. Saturated fats and trans fats contribute to total cholesterol and triglycerides in the body and eventually to cardiovascular disease and some cancers. Most fat should come from polyunsaturated sources such as vegetable oil and fish oil and monounsaturated sources such as canola oil, olive oil, or avocados. Ten percent or more of calories should come from monounsaturated sources.

The revised 2006 nutritional labels should list the kinds of fats in each product. However, if the amount of anything, including trans fats, is 0.5 mg or less per serving, the manufacturer can list it as not present. If a person chooses to have more than one serving of the product, the trans fats and other ingredients could add up. If "hydrogenated" is listed anywhere in the ingredients, trans fat is present.

Low-fat protein should make up the rest of the calories that we eat. Such items as lean meat, chicken, turkey, and ham as well as low- or no-fat dairy should be eaten every day. Vegetarians substitute vegetable protein from a variety of sources such as whole grains, legumes, vegetables, and starches as well as eggs and dairy products to meet their protein needs. For vegans, who eat no animal products, meeting their calcium, iron, and vitamin B-12 needs can be difficult, and their diets may need to be supplemented with a multivitamin and mineral source.

WEIGHT LOSS

Weight loss is recommended for anyone whose body mass index indicates that they are overweight or obese (see Figure 2.1). Even a small weight loss of 10–20 pounds can reverse insulin resistance and improve blood sugar. This might be a selling point to use with clients. Weight loss should be achieved over a period of time with a loss of 1–2 pounds per week. This can be achieved by portion control, decreasing intake of high-calorie foods and foods with empty calories, and increasing physical activity. Calories ingested must not exceed calories burned or weight gain will result. Caloric intake for most adults should not be less than 1,000–1,200 Kcal/day for women and 1,200–1,600 Kcal/day for men (ADA, 2006, p. S11). Anything less will result in a reprogramming of the rate at which calories are burned. Because the body thinks we are starving, the absorption of nutrients by the small intestine gets very efficient and our basal metabolic rate decreases to conserve energy. Thus when we increase calories after we have lost weight, we gain it right back and gain even more. It takes much more effort to increase our metabolic rate to burn more calories than to decrease it. Any caloric restriction below the recommended limits stated above will result in what many call yo-yo dieting and will be counterproductive.

One of the most useful tools to achieve weight loss is a dietary journal. Keeping track of everything eaten, the timing of meals and snacks,

FIGURE 2.1 BODY MASS INDEX

BMI is body weight in kilograms divided by height in meters squared. To calculate BMI using pounds and inches, perform the following steps:

1. Multiply weight in pounds by 703.
2. Multiply height in inches times itself.
3. Divide the results of step 1 by step 2 and compare with results below.

Example:

1. 170 pounds × 703 = 119,510.
2. 5 feet, 4 inches = 64 × 64 = 4,096
3. 119510 ÷ 4,096 = 29.177 = overweight (see below)

Disease risk based on BMI and waist circumference

Weight category	BMI	Waist circumference	
		≤ 40 in men ≤ 35 in women	> 40 in men > 35 in women
Underweight	< 18.5	Low	–
Normal weight	18.5–24.9	Low	–
Overweight	25–29.9	Increased	High
Obese	30–39.9	High	Very high
Morbidly obese	≥ 40	Very high	Extremely high

the amounts of each food item (which means measuring and weighing), to accurately calculate calories and grams of carbohydrates, protein, and fat, and any emotions that accompany eating patterns is very useful in generating an action plan to change and improve eating habits. Of course, physical activity is a part of any weight-loss program. In order to lose 1–2 pounds per week, we must decrease intake by 500–1,000 calories per day or burn that much by increasing physical activity or combine both modalities.

OLD FOOD PYRAMID VERSUS 2005 DIETARY GUIDELINES

The 2005 Dietary Guidelines for Americans developed by the U.S. Department of Agriculture (USDA) and the U.S. Department of Health and Human Services is an attempt to individualize the food pyramid. The Web site http://mypyramid.gov provides authoritative advice for anyone

2 years old and older concerning healthy dietary habits that reduce the risk of major chronic diseases. All anyone has to do is key in his or her age, gender, and physical activity level truthfully and a personalized dietary recommendation based on the 2005 guidelines is produced. It details the kinds and amounts of foods to eat each day and provides encouragement to improve dietary choices and make lifestyle changes in small incremental steps. "My Pyramid Tracker" provides a means to monitor a person's progress. Before nurses can truly understand how to help someone else to modify his or her diet and increase healthy choices, they need to go to this impressive site and see how their diet measures up to the recommendation for age, gender, and physical activity.

Thankfully, the diabetic (ADA) diets of the past are gone. What nurses need to remember is that the diet appropriate for a client with diabetes is a nutritious, well-balanced diet full of choices including sugar. It is a diet that meets all of the recommendations from the American Heart Association, the American Cancer Society, and the new 2005 Dietary Guidelines for Americans. It is full of vitamins, minerals, antioxidants, flavonoids, and other nutrients that everyone needs to stay healthy. Someone is always telling me that I cannot eat this or that because I have diabetes. My answer to them is usually, "If I cannot eat it, maybe you should not eat it." I might also add, "If I can give myself sufficient insulin to control blood sugar as your pancreas does, all that will happen is that we will both put on weight."

CARB COUNTING

If insulin administered should match the amount of carbohydrates ingested, then counting carbs is a worthwhile endeavor. The foods that have the greatest effect on blood sugar include the items in the bread/cereal food group, the fruit group, the milk group, and starchy vegetables like peas, corn, lima beans, potatoes, and dried or canned beans, and sweets, of course. The amount of each is also important. The following is a practical guide to counting grams of carbohydrates.

The bread/cereal/pasta group equals 15 grams of carbohydrates per serving

Bread	1 slice
Pasta	1/2 cup
Dry cereal	1 oz

Cooked cereal	1/2 cup
Starchy vegetables	1/3 to 1/2 cup (cooked)

The fruit group equals 15 grams of carbohydrates per serving

Fresh fruit	1 medium piece
Fruit juice	1/3 to 1/2 cup

The milk group equals 12 grams of carbohydrates per serving

Milk	1 cup
Yogurt, plain	3/4 cup

Nonstarchy vegetables have 5 grams of carbohydrates per 1/2 cup cooked or 1 cup raw. Meats and fats have no carbohydrates unless cooked or mixed with something that does. Counting carbs has gotten much easier with food labels being so well marked. A serving size is at the top of the food label. If a serving size is doubled, the carb grams, as well as all other entities on the label, must be doubled.

Fiber is a carbohydrate. However, it is hard to digest and absorb. Most authorities advise to subtract the fiber grams if the total for the meal exceeds 5 grams. The USDA advises the healthy American to have at least 25 grams of fiber per day for good colon health, so looking for foods that are good sources of fiber is a fruitful endeavor. Breads should have at least 3 grams of fiber per slice (some labels list serving size as 2 slices, so fiber content should be halved). Dry cereals should have at least 5 grams of fiber per 1 ounce serving to be a good source. Reading labels to find the fiber grams is a must in order to count carbs accurately. Fruits with eatable skins are good sources of fiber, as are raw vegetables.

According to Warshaw and Boderman, "Carbohydrates begin to raise blood glucose within 15 minutes after initiation of food intake and are converted to nearly 100% glucose within 2 hours…. The ADA nutrition recommendations encourage a focus on total carbohydrate intake rather than differentiating between types of carbohydrates" (Warshaw & Boderman, 2001, p. 1).

ALCOHOL: PROS AND CONS

Many people think that anyone with diabetes should not drink alcoholic beverages. Clients may ask the nurse, and so you need to know what to tell them. Studies have shown that moderate drinking, no more than one to two drinks per day, can reduce the risk of heart disease by 30–50% by increasing the HDL cholesterol levels and preventing clot formation in the arteries (Wilder, Cheskin, & Margolis, 2006). Johns Hopkins White Papers: Nutrition and Weight Control for Longevity (2006) lists the following recommendations with regard to alcohol:

1. If you currently don't drink alcohol, do not start.
2. If you are a man, limit yourself to one to two drinks per day and cut this in half if over the age of 65. It takes longer to detoxify alcohol.
3. If you are a woman, limit intake to no more than one drink per day and take half that amount if over 65.
4. Heavy alcohol consumption (defined as more than two drinks per day) can cause or worsen hypertension, cardiovascular disease, and liver disease.
5. Alcohol can interfere with many medications.

Alcohol can be part of the diet for a person with diabetes as long as it is used in moderation and the calories and carbohydrates are accounted for. Alcohol delivers 7 calories per gram and is metabolized like a fat. One drink is defined as a 12-ounce beer, 5 ounces of wine, or 1.5 ounces of distilled spirits. Alcohol can cause hypoglycemia, so it should be consumed with food. If hypoglycemia occurs, alcohol prevents the liver from responding to glucagon, so blood sugar may drop dangerously low. Because the behavior of someone experiencing hypoglycemia is often mistaken for drunkenness, a diabetic with alcohol on his or her breath may not be treated appropriately, potentially resulting in brain damage and even death from severe hypoglycemia.

SICK-DAY MANAGEMENT

This is one of the most important pieces if information for someone with diabetes to know in order to prevent further illness from hypo-or hyperglycemia. Testing blood sugar every 2–4 hours is a must. If a blood sugar is high, clients must stay hydrated with diet or noncaloric drinks such as water, broth, sugar-free tea or coffee, and sugar-free gelatin or popsicles.

If a blood sugar is normal or low, then regular cola or fruit drinks need to be consumed. Start drinking fluids slowly 1–2 hours after vomiting or diarrhea. If insulin or a secretagogue medication has already been administered, glucose tablets or gels should be available to prevent or treat hypoglycemia.

Medical nutrition management for clients with diabetes can be an adventure in good health for the whole family if approached in a positive manner. Since my diagnosis, my whole family has benefited from a healthy diet because I never prepare anything I should not eat. The emphasis should be on making changes gradually and keeping some favorite foods for eating sporadically in the diet.

REFERENCES

American Diabetes Association. (2006). ADA 2006 Standards of medical care in diabetes—2006. *Diabetes Care, 29*, S4–S42.

U.S. Department of Agriculture. (2005). The 2005 dietary guidelines for Americans. Retrieved July 13, 2005, from http://mypyramid.gov

Warshaw, H. S., & Boderman, K. M. (2001). Practical carbohydrate counting. Alexandria, VA: American Diabetes Association.

Wilder, L. B., Cheskin, L. J., & Margolis, S. (2006). Johns Hopkins white papers: Nutrition and weight control for longevity. Redding, CT: Medletter Associates.

3

Treatment: Physical Activity

What can be done at ANYTIME, will be done at NO TIME.

Old Scottish Proverb

I have decided to use the term *physical activity* interchangeably with *exercise* because exercise also has a negative connotation for many people. Just like *diet*, *exercise* seems to portray punishing athletic endeavors: long, boring, and sweaty walking, running, or weight lifting at the gym. Physical activity, on the other hand, means physical movement, the kind that gets you out of bed in the morning and moving throughout the day. It is important to remind ourselves that it all counts toward keeping our muscles toned and our bones strong. What we all need is more of it.

I was in Chicago recently, visiting my daughter, and was amazed to see fewer obese children and adults than in my own smaller city of Richmond, Virginia. The population in this and, I presume, other large cities is very dense with most people living in high-rise apartments and condos. Space to park a car is at a premium, and gas prices are horrific. Most Chicagoans walk to stores, restaurants, friends' homes, or at least to the closest mass transit facility. During my visit we ate out a lot, but I lost weight. What a refreshing turn of events! As a result, I am now walking from my home to anywhere that is a mile or so away instead of always getting in my car. Of course, this is pending inclement weather, but my experience in Chicago has increased the amount of walking that I do. As nurses, we must be able to give evidence that we take our own advice seriously.

BENEFITS OF EXERCISE

The benefits of physical activity are numerous and well documented. Physical activity has the following effects:

- helps to control weight by increasing muscle tissue and decreasing fat production because the calories consumed are burned more efficiently by the body. Increased muscle mass (lean tissue) increases basal metabolic rate even at rest so more calories are burned all day long and even while sleeping.
- increases the efficiency of the heart and lungs by increasing demands on their functions, thus exercising the heart muscle and increasing the depth of respirations needed to sustain aerobic activity. This decreases resting heart rate and respiratory rate.
- improves digestion and elimination in the gastrointestinal tract by increasing peristalsis and blood flow to the stomach and intestines.
- improves blood pressure, blood flow, and cholesterol levels by causing vasodilation of blood vessels, increasing HDL (the good cholesterol), and decreasing LDL (the bad cholesterol) and triglycerides (Saudek & Margolis, 2006).
- improves sleep patterns by increasing blood flow to muscles and thus removing lactic acid buildup. Strenuous exercise should not be done within 3 hours of sleep time, however, because lactic acid may remain in muscles causing stiffness and pain.
- increases a sense of well-being by providing a productive means of getting rid of excess negative emotions such as anxiety, anger, frustration, and so forth, and increasing positive feelings of empowerment and pride in accomplishing a set goal.

If the above is not incentive enough for clients with diabetes, add the fact that physical activity helps to lower blood sugar. Because physical activity makes muscle more sensitive to insulin, glucose is used at a much faster rate. So what is not to like about increased physical activity?

Tips to help fit in a more active lifestyle include

- getting up earlier to go for a run, a walk, or a bike ride. In fact, why not watch or listen to the morning news while riding your stationary bike?
- eating dinner a little earlier to fit in some exercise before relaxing for the day
- using part of a lunch break to walk or exercise
- joining a gym or a neighborhood sports team. Athletic talent is not usually required.

- running or walking around an inside or outside track on the way home from work
- exercising a dog or actively playing with children or grandchildren
- vacuuming, cleaning tile in a bathroom, scrubbing floors, or performing other chores. These are very productive activities even if not the most fun things to do. Listening to music or an audio book can make the time fly by.
- performing any physical activity that you find appealing and worth your time and energy.

Making it a daily routine is as important as going to work or getting to an appointment. Make it a family affair and get the kids active and away from the TV or computer. If an incentive to set a specific time for physical activity is needed, reread the Scottish proverb at the beginning of this chapter.

POTENTIAL PROBLEMS WITH EXERCISE

There *is* a downside to physical activity for anyone on insulin or oral medications that make the pancreas secrete more insulin. The problem is hypoglycemia. Tell clients that low blood sugar can be avoided, however, by adhering to the following advice:

1. The best time to be active is about 30 minutes to 1 hour after a meal. I know what your mother always told you, but unless the activity is prolonged (more than 60 minutes) or very strenuous (swimming 50 laps of an Olympic-size pool) or your meal is loaded with fats and protein (10-ounce steak, large order of fries), you will not get abdominal cramps.
2. When exercise occurs more than 2 hours after eating, a blood sugar check is in order. If it is less than 120 mg/dl, consider eating or drinking something that has about 15–30 mg of carbohydrates, such as a piece of fruit, 6 ounces of orange juice, or an 8-ounce glass of milk. It might be better to take less insulin prior to a meal that precedes planned exercise.

   If blood sugar is over 250 mg/dl or especially over 350 mg/dl, check urine for ketones, and postpone exercise until blood sugar is less than 250 mg/dl and ketonuria is gone. Taking rapid-acting insulin and waiting 30 minutes or so should help (Scheiner, 2004).

When blood sugar is high, it means that the body does not have enough insulin to keep it in normal range by helping the blood glucose to enter cells. This includes muscle cells, which store glucose as glycogen. When muscle cells are not fed glucose to perform physical activity, they dump stored glycogen into the blood so these muscle cells can burn this glucose. Unfortunately, this use of glucose does not happen because there is insufficient insulin to transport the blood sugar into muscle cells. The end result after exercising with high blood sugar can be even higher blood sugar and a very sluggish feeling. When cells cannot get to glucose, fat is burned for energy, resulting in blood and urine ketones.

3. Always carry glucose tablets when taking insulin or oral medications that increase pancreatic secretions. If hypoglycemia unawareness is a problem, exercise with someone who is aware of symptoms and can get help if the need should arise.

4. If insulin injections are used, avoid injecting into fatty areas of extremities used during exercise. This really means that if brisk walking, jogging, swimming, or skiing are involved, avoid giving insulin in upper thighs and buttocks. If lifting weights or heavy housecleaning is anticipated, avoid the back of upper arms. Exercise increases blood supply to active muscles, which causes vasodilatation to smaller blood vessels in the subcutaneous fatty layer directly above the muscles. If insulin has been injected there, it will be absorbed into the bloodstream much faster than anticipated. This, along with the fact that exercise increases insulin sensitivity of muscles and other tissue, makes hypoglycemia more likely.

5. Check blood sugar a couple of hours after exercising, because an intense workout may cause hypoglycemia for several hours. Making the body more insulin sensitive has its drawbacks if the usual amount of insulin or oral agent is taken and exercise is added. It may be wise to discuss with a doctor decreasing medication on days when planned exercise is prolonged and/or strenuous in order to prevent hypoglycemia (Scheiner, 2004).

6. Before starting an exercise program, check with a physician who may order an exercise stress test to see how the heart and blood pressure respond. If diabetic complications are part of the picture, see Table 3.1 for common restrictions.

TABLE 3.1 Diabetic Complications and Exercise

Complications	Exercise to avoid	Rationale	Choose instead
Peripheral neuropathy	Jogging Brisk walking Climbing	May cause foot trauma, turned ankle, falls	Swimming Stationary bike Rowing machine
Autonomic neuropathy	Strenuous or prolonged exercise	Decreased cardiovascular response, postural hypotension	Walking Swimming Treadmill
Proliferative retinopathy	Jogging Skiing Body contact sports Any jarring or rapid head movement Heavy lifting Any use of Valsalva breath holding	May cause retinal detachment or vitreous hemorrhage	Walking Swimming Stationary bike
Nephropathy	Strenuous or prolonged exercise	May increase proteinuria Does not affect progression of renal disease	Walking Swimming Exercise equipment for mild to moderate intensity and duration
Cardiovascular disease including congestive heart failure (CHF) and hypertension	Heavy lifting Any use of Valsalva breath holding Strenuous or prolonged exercise	May cause angina, arrhythmias, and increased blood pressure if not well controlled	Swimming Treadmill Stationary bike

7. Adequate hydration is important for everyone, whether they exercise or not. However, it is extremely important for all to drink water before and after exercising. If physical activity is very strenuous or prolonged, fluid intake during exercise is important to prevent dehydration from excessive perspiration. Water is the best choice for fluid replacement. Sports drinks contain calories, sugar, and electrolytes, which are usually only needed by endurance athletes.

8. Inspect feet after exercise to check for blisters and/or reddened areas. This is especially important for those with peripheral neuropathy or with peripheral vascular disease who may not feel an injury. Adequate circulation is needed to heal and prevent infection even with a minor wound. Any injured skin and tissue should be reported to a physician immediately.

9. It goes without saying that good supportive shoes and comfortable clothing are a must. Checking the inside of shoes for worn areas or small items that may cause discomfort or injury is important for everyone. My nondiabetic husband once realized his foot was sharing a shoe with an insect and now always looks before sliding his feet into shoes.

People with diabetes need to be reminded that healthy lifestyle choices are a must for everyone and not an imposition as a result of having diabetes. Physical activity is important for persons of any age. All adults should try to achieve the recommended 10,000 steps a day. Inexpensive step counters and aerobic monitors are easily found in drug and variety stores. Recording activity level is both empowering and motivating. Some monitors equate steps taken with calories burned and miles walked. Because every step counts, a step counter may provide the encouragement to take the stairs instead of the elevator or to walk to do errands. Giving examples of how physical activity impacts *our* life can be the incentive a client needs to *just do it!*

REFERENCES

Saudek, C. D., & Margolis, S. (2006). *Johns Hopkins white papers: Diabetes.* Redding, CT: Medletter Associates.

Scheiner, G. (2004). *Think like a pancreas.* New York: Marlowe & Company.

4

Treatment: Medication

A man too busy to take care of his health is like a mechanic too busy to take care of his tools.

Spanish Proverb

When lifestyle changes like healthy eating, weight loss, and exercise are not enough to normalize blood sugars, there is always medication. The classifications of oral agents and types of insulin have expanded exponentially in the last 10 years. Diabetes is big business, and pharmaceutical companies are leading the pack to cash in. Besides new medications, we now have combinations of medications that complement each other in one pill. So much has happened so quickly that it is confusing and difficult for health care professionals to keep up. By the time you read this, there will be newer, more powerful, and useful drugs on the market. As each drug is discussed, the Web address of the drug and the company that makes it will be listed so you can do further research. It will be several years before all of the new drugs go off patent and their generic equivalents are available. That means that the newest and often best medications are very expensive. Many of the pharmaceutical companies have programs for providing their new drugs for free or at reduced cost to clients who meet certain criteria. So if a client can no longer afford the necessary medications, refer him or her to one of the following Web sites:

1. Partnership for Prescription Assistance, http://www.PPARx.org, 1-888-4PPA-NOW (477-2669)
2. National Diabetes Information Clearing House (NDIC), http://diabetes.niddk.nih.gov/dm/pubs/financialhelp/

Clients must be referred through their physician, but letting a client know this service exists may start the ball rolling. In addition, Googling (http://www.google.com) any new drug trade name will result in a list of Web sites with information for patients and health care professionals.

ORAL ANTIDIABETIC MEDICATIONS

Secretagogues

Secretagogues are drugs that induce the pancreas to increase its production of insulin. Three classes of secretagogues are currently in use. These include sulfonylureas, meglitinides, and D-phenylalanine derivatives. Because they all work a little differently, they will be discussed separately (see Table 4.1.)

Sulfonylureas

Sulfonylureas were the first and only oral antidiabetic drugs for type 2 diabetics for many years. The only first-generation sulfonylurea still on the market is Diabinese. As you can see in Table 4.1, second-generation drugs are more potent so can be given at lower dosages. They also have fewer side effects than the first-generation drugs, although hypoglycemia is still a possibility when meals are omitted or delayed or exercise is prolonged. They may also cause weight gain, water retention, and sometimes flushing with alcohol, although this is less common than with Diabinese. The weight gain is an especially vexing problem, as increased weight increases insulin resistance. Water retention can also increase blood pressure, which is often a part of the diabetic picture. Sulfonylureas should only be prescribed for type 2 clients who are able to increase their beta cell production of insulin. Because type 2 diabetes is a progressive disease, eventually the beta cells will have no more to give, and different drugs, including insulin, may be added or substituted to bring blood glucose into normal range. Sulfonylureas are also mild sulfa drugs that may not be appropriate for anyone with an allergy to sulfa. The following is a list of newer sulfonylureas along with the names of the companies that manufacture them and the Web URLs for more information. Starred drugs are now available as generics.

Glucotrol* and Glucatrol XL*	Pfizer Inc.	http://www.pfizer.com/pfizer/do/medicines/mn_glucotrol_xl.jsp
DiaBeta*	Sanofi-Aventis US	http://products.sanofi-aventis.us/diabeta/diabeta.html

TABLE 4.1 Oral Antidiabetic Medication

Generic name	Trade name	Usual dose	Directions	Peak	Duration	Target organ	Comments
Sulfonylureas							
First generation							
- chlorpropamide	Diabinese*	250–500 mg	Take with breakfast	2–4 hrs	24–28 hrs	Pancreas	All: May be used alone or in combination with metformin, thiazolidinediones, and alpha-glucosidase inhibitors. Hypoglycemia may be prolonged. May cause water retention, weight gain. With alcohol may cause flushing.
Second generation							
- glipizide	Glucatrol*	5–40 mg	1–2x/day AC meal	1–3 hrs	12–24 hrs	Pancreas	
	Glucatrol XL*	5–20 mg	Take with breakfast	6–12 hrs	24 hrs		
- glyburide	DiaBeta*	5–20 mg	1–2x/day AC meal	2–4 hrs	24 hrs		
	Glynase PresTab	6–20 mg	1–2x/day AC meal	2–4 hrs	24 hrs		
	Micronase		1–2x/day AC meal	2–4 hrs	24 hrs		
- glimeperide	Amaryl	5–12 mg 2–8 mg	Take with breakfast	2–3 hrs	24 hrs		
Meglitinides							
- repaglinide	Prandin	0.5–2 mg	Take before meals	1 hr	2–4 hrs	Pancreas	Alone or in combination with other nonsecretagogues. Less chance of hypoglycemia.
D-phenylalanine derivatives							
- nateglinide	Starlix	60–120 mg	Take before meals	1–2 hrs	2–3 hrs	Pancreas	Alone or in combination with other nonsecretagogues. Less chance of hypoglycemia.

(continued)

TABLE 4.1 *(continued)*

Generic name	Trade name	Usual dose	Directions	Peak	Duration	Target organ	Comments
Biguanides							
- metformin	Glucophage*	500 mg	2–3x/day AC meals		12 hrs	Liver and muscles	Used alone, no weight gain or hypoglycemia. May be used with all other classes of antidiabetic drugs including insulin.
	Glucophage XR	500 mg	Take with PM meal		24 hrs		
	Glumetza	500 mg	Take with PM meal		24 hrs		
- metformin (liquid)	Riomet	500 mg/5 ml	Take 5 ml daily		24 hrs		
Thiazolidinediones							
pioglitazone	Actos	15 mg	1–2x/day with or without meals	3 hrs	16–34 hrs	Muscles	May be used with all other classes of antidiabetic drugs including insulin.
rosiglitazone	Avandia	4 mg					
Alpha-glucosidase inhibitors							
acarbose	Precose*	50 mg	Take just before eating	rapid	1 hr	Small intestines	May be used with all other classes of antidiabetic drugs including insulin. Causes gas and bloating.
miglitol	Glyset	50 mg					
Combination agents							
- glipizide/metformin	Metaglip	5 mg/500 mg	Take with meals	See each drug	See separate drugs	See separate drugs	See separate drugs
- glyburide/metformin	Glucovance	5 mg/500 mg	Take with meals				
- rosiglitazone/metformin	Avandamet	4 mg/500 mg	Take with meals				

*Available as a generic

Glynase PresTab	Pfizer Inc.	http://www.pfizer.com/pfizer/download/ uspi_glynase.pdf
Micronase	Pfizer Inc.	http://www.pfizer.com/pfizer/download/ uspi_micronase.pdf
Amaryl	Sanofi-Aventis US	http://products.sanofi-aventis.us/ index.html

Meglitinides

The only drug approved by the FDA to date in this class is repaglinide (Prandin). Its mechanism of action is similar to sulfonylureas; however, it acts much more rapidly. Therefore, it is taken right before a meal and increases insulin production dependent on blood glucose from this meal. This increases the flexibility of meal planning and decreases incidence of hypoglycemia because it is not taken unless a meal is to be eaten within 30 minutes. It can be taken alone or combined with metformin, alpha-glucosidase inhibitors, or thiazolidinediones.

| Prandin | Novo Nordisk, Inc. | http://www.prandin. com/ |

D-Phenylalanine Derivatives

The only FDA-approved drug in this class is nateglinide (Starlix). This drug acts similarly to Prandin in that it stimulates a rapid release of insulin from the beta cells thus controlling blood sugars after meals. It is taken right before a meal, so the side effect of hypoglycemia is rare. Because it is metabolized and partially excreted by the liver, its duration of action can be prolonged in people with significant liver disease, resulting in an increased the risk of hypoglycemia. This drug can be taken alone or in combination with metformin to enhance insulin sensitivity.

| Starlix | Novartis Pharmaceuticals USA | http://www.starlix.com/ index.jsp |

Biguanides

Drugs in this class act primarily to decrease the liver's inappropriate release of glycogen into the blood, thus increasing blood sugar. It also improves cellular insulin sensitivity, both problems in type 2 diabetes.

Metformin (Glucophage) was the first nonsulfonylurea to be added to the arsenal of oral agents for type 2 diabetes. Side effects include diarrhea, bloating, and nausea, all of which decrease over time and are minimized by taking the lowest dose and titrating upward until glycemic control is achieved. The most problematic adverse effect is lactic acidosis, which is rare, but can be fatal. Clients with liver or renal disease should not take this drug. When taken alone, Glucophage does not contribute to weight gain or cause hypoglycemia. It may even lower LDL cholesterol (bad cholesterol) and triglyceride levels, which are both problems in type 2 diabetes. This drug can be used as a first-line agent to improve glycemic control, or it can be combined with sulfonylureas, meglitinides (Prandin), alpha-glucosidase inhibitors (Precose and Glyset), thiazolidinediones (Actos and Avandia), and insulin. Three combination pills are currently available: Glucovance (metformin and glyburide), Metaglip (metformin and glipizide), and Avandamet (metformin and rosiglitazone). As the rate of type 2 diabetes increases, more drug companies will add to the available combinations. Combination drugs increase ease of use and compliance as well as cost. The two separate medications may currently both be available as generics, but the new combination will not be available as a generic for several years. A new drug in this class, Glumetza, an extended-release formulation of metformin codeveloped by Biovail and Depomed, Inc., and now distributed by Depomed, Inc., for the treatment of type 2 diabetes, received FDA approval in June 2005. It is a metformin derivative that may have fewer side effects than metformin. Riomet by Ranbaxy Laboratories, Inc., is a liquid formulation of metformin.

Glucophage and Glucophage XR	Bristol-Myers Squibb Company	http://www.glucophagexr.com/ landing/data/index.html
Glumetza	Depomed Inc.	http://www.depomedinc.com/ products_glumetza.htm
Riomet	Ranbaxy Laboratories, Inc.	http://www.riomet.com
Glucovance	Bristol-Myers Squibb Company	http://www.glucovance.com/ products/data/index.html
Avandamet	GlaxoSmithKline	http://www.avandia.com/about_ avandamet/avandamet.html

Metaglip   Bristol-Myers   http://www.metaglip.com/landing/
              Squibb Company   data/index.html

Thiazolidinediones

This group of drugs, better known as "glitazones," includes pioglitazone (Actos) and rosiglitazone (Avandia). They act by decreasing cellular resistance to insulin, thus improving control of blood sugars. The obese population of type 2 diabetics may improve glycemic control by adding one of these drug to lifestyle changes of weight loss, healthy diet, and increased physical activity. It can also be taken with sulfonylureas, meglitinides (Prandin), metformin (Glucophage or as Avandamet), alpha-glucosidase inhibitors (Precose or Glyset), or insulin. The FDA recommends liver function tests be done before and during treatment with this class of drugs because the first one, troglitazon (Rezulin), was withdrawn from the market in 2000 due to reports of rare incidents of liver failure and related deaths. The two newer drugs, Actos and Avandia, are much less toxic to the liver, but patient selection must be appropriate. If a patient's liver enzymes increase, the drug is usually discontinued for this individual.

Glitazone drugs can also cause fluid retention and rapid weight gain independent of fluid retention. Clients at risk for congestive heart failure should probably not take this drug. All clients taking these drugs need to be monitored for cardiac function and weight gain, ruling out fluid retention as the cause.

Because many clients with type 2 diabetes also may be taking drugs to lower cholesterol, the name of their antihyperlipidemic should be documented. Cholestyramine (Questran) inhibits the absorption of glitazones as well as other drugs and should not be taken at the same time. It may take several weeks or months to see the full effect of Actos or Avandia, so blood sugars should be monitored closely. If insulin or a secretagogue is taken during this time, the dose may need to be lowered as the glitazone kicks in. A new combination drug called Avandadryl is on the market. This drug combines Avandia and glimeperide, a sulfonyl-urea (trade name Amaryl). It has the same precautions concerning liver function that all glitazones have and should be administered with the first good meal of the day to minimize hypoglycemia from Amaryl.

Actos	Takeda Pharmaceuticals North America, Inc., and Eli Lilly and Company	http://www.actos.com/index.asp
Avandia	GlaxoSmithKline	http://www.avandia.com/
Avandadryl	GlaxoSmithKline	http://www.avandia.com/about_ avandaryl/avandaryl.html

Alpha-Glucosidase Inhibitors

The two drugs in this class, acarbose (Precose; called Glucobay in Europe and Prandase in Canada) and miglitol (Glyset), work in the small intestine to delay the digestion of carbohydrates (starches and sucrose) and decrease the peak postprandial (after meal) glucose levels allowing insulin production to better match glucose absorption. They can be taken alone or in combination with sulfonylureas, repaglinide (Prandin), metformin (Glucophage), thiazolidinediones (Actos or Avandia), or insulin. When taken alone, these drugs do not cause hypoglycemia, but when taken with other agents that do cause low blood sugar, only glucose (as in glucose tablets or gel) or fructose from fruit juice will treat the hypoglycemia.

The most common side effects are gas, diarrhea, and cramps. These diminish with time and are minimized by starting at the lowest dose and gradually increasing it if needed to control blood sugars. Because of these side effects, this drug may not be appropriate for anyone with irritable bowel syndrome.

| Precose* | Bayer HealthCare | http://www.precose.com/en/ professional/facts/index.html |
| Glyset | Pfizer, Inc. | http://www.pfizer.com/pfizer/do/ medicines/mn_uspi.jsp |

INJECTABLE ANTIDIABETIC MEDICATION

Insulin

The body needs insulin 24/7. When the islet cells of the pancreas perform as intended, a small amount of endogenous (originating from within the body) insulin is secreted constantly to allow some glucose to enter cells for cellular function. When we inject exogenous (originating outside the body) insulin for this purpose, we refer to it as a basal insulin. As the normal islet cells sense a rise in blood sugar from a meal or snack, the beta cells produce more endogenous insulin to keep blood sugar within the normal range. We can give bolus doses of exogenous insulin prior to eating to mimic this activity when pancreatic function is compromised. The purposes of insulin therapy are (1) to maximize glycemic control while minimizing the risk of hypoglycemia, and (2) to effectively mimic the body's physiologic need for insulin as both basal and bolus rates.

Tight glycemic control, especially using insulin, has been shown in several clinical trials to prevent or delay the onset of complications caused by hyperglycemia. The unintended consequence of keeping blood sugars at near-normal levels is hypoglycemia. The pancreas, when it is healthy, does a much better job at doing this than the human brain, even aided by a glucose meter and multiple insulin injections or the use of an insulin pump. However, with effort and the right combination of insulins, clients with type 1 and type 2 diabetes can achieve close to normal glycemic control as measured by hemoglobin A_{1c} with minimal hypoglycemic events.

Obviously, all type 1 diabetics take a basal insulin that keeps their body functioning between meals and throughout the night and a bolus insulin dose before meals. Basal insulins can be comprised of

1. one dose per day of a long-acting insulin,
2. two doses of an intermediate-acting insulin, or
3. various basal rates with rapid-acting insulin using an insulin pump.

Bolus doses of insulin to cover episodes of hyperglycemia and meal or snack carbohydrate amounts are given as needed. This is much easier to do with an insulin pump, but it also can be managed by giving injections of rapid-acting insulin prior to a meal or snack. Additional insulin can be added or subtracted based on the current blood sugar level. For instance, a person might start with a sliding scale for rapid-acting insulin to take care of higher-than-normal blood sugar prior to meals.

A set ratio of units of insulin to grams of carbohydrates (see "Carb Counting" in chapter 2) would be added to the sliding scale amount to minimize the effect of the meal or snack on blood sugar. Examples of insulin to carbohydrate ratios might resemble the following:

1 unit of insulin for every 10 grams of carbohydrate
1 unit of insulin for every 12 grams of carbohydrate
1 unit of insulin for every 15 grams of carbohydrate
1 unit of insulin for every 20 grams of carbohydrate

This ratio may be different at each meal or may remain the same. If this sounds difficult, it is. The troubling aspect of working all of this out is that each person responds to food and insulin differently, so it is a matter of trial and error. Because each person is different, a client has to be self-reliant and willing to experiment. Only those committed to their long-term survival and desire to live as normal a life as possible will be able to handle this challenge.

Insulin therapy for clients with type 2 diabetes is gaining more interest. Because hyperglycemia has such devastating consequences over time, glycemic control needs to be achieved as soon as possible. Insulin is not used as a last resort with type 2 diabetics or as an indication that all attempts with oral agents have failed. It should never be used as a threat or punishment for people who are *noncompliant* with weight loss, proper nutrition, and increase in physical activity. It may be the treatment of choice for some clients with type 2 diabetes. Insulin should be used in treating type 2 diabetes when

1. hyperglycemia is severe at diagnosis,
2. glycemic control is not achieved with lifestyle changes and combinations of oral meds,
3. uncontrolled hyperglycemia is caused by infection, acute injury, surgery, heart attack, stroke, or other cardiovascular incident,
4. the above incidents cause ketonemia and/or ketonuria and uncontrolled weight loss,
5. liver and/or renal disease complicate metabolism and excretion of oral antidiabetic medications, or
6. pregnancy is a contraindication to the use of some oral antidiabetic drugs. (ADA, 2003)

The American Diabetes Association recommends that the use of insulin be viewed in the same light as all oral agents for those with type 2 diabetes and that more clients be started on insulin alone or in combination with metformin or other nonsecretagogues sooner rather than later (ADA, 2003).

If glycemic control is delayed, the risk of developing chronic complications is increased. The sooner blood sugars are controlled, the better.

Types of Insulin

Insulin was discovered in the 1920s and consisted of a short-acting insulin distillate from the pancreas of dogs. Children with type 1 diabetes needed four or five injections per day, even during the night. In the 1940s, protamine was added to regular insulin to make NPH (protomine hagedorn) insulin and zinc was added to regular insulin to make lente insulin. This slowed the onset, peak, and, most importantly, duration of insulin and decreased the number of injections per day. Most insulin used today in the United States is manufactured in a lab using recombinant DNA technology. Prior to 1985, insulin came from the pancreases of cows and pigs and was marketed as beef, beef-pork, or purified porcine insulin. Porcine insulin was the closest in molecular structure to endogenous human insulin. The use of insulin from different species gave rise to allergic reactions, immunologic suppression of this insulin's action, and the fear that there would not be sufficient animal pancreases to meet the increasing need for insulin therapy. The new rapid-acting insulin analogs have had a huge impact on controlling postmeal hyperglycemia and/or hypoglycemia. If enough regular insulin is given to keep 2-hour postprandial blood sugar under 140 mg/dl, it would often cause a low blood sugar 3–4 hours later. The minimum 30-minute delay in eating after the insulin dose is often a problem as well. See Table 4.2 for a list of the types of insulin and their properties. Regular insulin, although the shortest acting insulin we had for decades, just does not match the increase in blood sugar generated by a typical meal. Its duration of action is also too long, causing frequent between-meal hypoglycemic reactions. To mimic the around-the-clock action of the body's insulin, intermediate and long-acting insulins were developed as previously described. Until 2005, NPH, lente, and ultralente insulins were available from both major companies that manufacture insulin in the United States. Eli Lilly and Novo Nordisk have stopped making lente and ultralente since the rapid and long-acting insulin analogs have supplanted their use. Each company also makes combination vials of NPH and regular human insulins for use in syringes and with their cartridge-filled pens. To learn more about the various types of human insulin currently on the market, visit the following Web sites.

TABLE 4.2 Types of Insulin

Type	Trade name	Onset	Peak	Duration	Comments
Rapid-acting					
- insulin lispro - insulin aspart	Humalog NovoLog	5–15 mins	30–90 mins	3–5 hrs	All: Prescription required. Inject before each meal. May be mixed with intermediate-acting insulin.
- insulin glulisine	Apidra				Apidra FDA approved April 2004
- inhaled Insulin	Exubera	30 min	108 min	6 hrs	Exubera FDA approved February 2006.
Short-acting					
- regular insulin	Humulin R Humulin R pen Novolin R Novolin R PenFill	30–60 mins	2–3 hrs	5–8 hrs	All: Inject 30 minutes before meals. May be mixed with intermediate-acting insulin.
Intermediate-acting					
- NPH insulin	Humulin N Humulin N pen Novolin N Novolin N PenFill	2–4 hrs	4–10 hrs	10–16 hrs	All: May be mixed with rapid or short-acting insulins.

Long-acting insulin - insulin glargine - insulin detemir	Lantus Levemir	2–4 hrs	None	20–24 hrs	Prescription required. Can not be mixed with other insulins.
Mixtures - 50% NPH/50% R - 70% NPH/30% R	Humulin 50/50 Humulin 70/30 Novolin 70/30 Novolin 70/30 PenFill Novolin 70/30 InnoLet	30–60 mins 30–60 mins 30–60 mins 30–60 mins	Dual Dual Dual Dual	10–16 hrs 10–16 hrs 10–16 hrs 10–16 hrs	Very convenient and useful for those with difficulty mixing insulins in same syringe.
- 70% aspart protamine/30% aspart	NovoLog 70/30 FlexPen	5–15 mins	Dual	10–16 hrs	Prescription required.
- 75% lispro protamine/25% lispro	Humalog Mix 75/25	5–15 mins	Dual	10–16 hrs	Prescription required.

Humulin R, N	Eli Lilly and Company	http://www.lillydiabetes. com/product/humulin_family. jsp?reqNavId=5.3
Humulin 70/30		
Humulin 50/50		
Humulin R, N, and 70/30 disposable, prefilled pens		
Novolin R, N and	Novo Nordisk US	http://www.insulindevice.com/ novopen/faq.asp
Novolin R, N and 70/30 Penfill		

Insulin Analogs

Insulin analogs are not human insulin. They are better. By rearranging some amino acids on human insulin's protein molecular structure, a faster onset and peak and shortened duration can be achieved. The result is an insulin that more closely matches the rise of blood sugar caused by a meal or snack. There are two insulin analogs in current use: insulin lispro (Humalog) and insulin aspart (Novolog), both of which are used for bolus dosing. Both can be used in insulin pumps or combined in a syringe with intermediate-acting NPH insulin for basal coverage. The third and newest rapid-onset insulin analog, insulin glulisine (Apidra), was approved by the FDA in April 2004. All rapid-acting insulin analogs can be used by type 1 and type 2 diabetics and injected or administered via insulin pump. All insulin analogs require a prescription and client education in their use, especially if the client has experience with short-acting regular insulin. Regular and NPH insulins as well as their various combinations do not require a prescription, although for health insurance coverage, one may be needed. Some states require that a person sign for insulin sold without a prescription to provide a record.

If rearranging amino acids can accelerate the action of human insulin, why can't different arrangements prolong the action? The first truly long-acting basal insulin was made by doing just that a few years ago. We now have two such basal insulins, insulin glargine (Lantus), and, the latest, insulin detemir (Levemir). These analogs are described as "peakless" and may be used with rapid- or short-acting insulin in treating type 1 and type 2 diabetes. They may also be used as a basal insulin with secretagogues or other oral agents for type 2 glycemic control. Both Lantus and Levemir require a prescription. Clients must be taught NOT to mix them with other insulins in the same syringe. A client must be willing to give two separate injections when using a basal insulin in conjunction with rapid- or short-acting insulin. Both types of insulin may, however, be given at the same time but in separate syringes. Both insulin glargine and insulin detemir improve fasting blood sugars and reduce the variability of peak action association with ultralente and intermediate-acting insulins. They can both be administered to children as young as 6 years old with type 1 diabetes.

Eli Lilly makes a premixed insulin, Humalog Mix 75/25, with 75% lispro protamine suspension and 25% insulin lispro. Novo Nordisk's premixed insulin, NovoLog 70/30, contains 70% aspart protamine and 30% insulin aspart. Both are available in vials for syringe use and cartridges for each company's insulin pens manufactured for client convenience. See each company's Web site below for more information about the mixtures and the insulin pens.

Humalog	Eli Lilly and Company	http://www.lillydiabetes.com/product/humalog.jsp?reqNavId=5.1
Humalog 75/25		
Humalog and Humalog 75/25 Prefilled Pen		http://www.lillydiabetes.com/product/insulin_pens.jsp?reqNavId=5.8
NovoLog	Novo Nordisk US	http://www.novolog.com/
NovoLog 70/30		http://www.novologmix70-30.com/homepage/
NovoLog Flexpen		http://www.novolog.com/consumer/devices/flexpen.asp
Apidra	Sonofi-Aventis US	http://www.apidra.com/
Lantus	Sonofi-Aventis US	http://www.lantus.com/consumer/index.do
Levemir	Novo Nordisk US	http://www.levemir-us.com/
Levemir Flexpen		http://www.insulindevice.com/lev_flexpen

Insulin Pumps

Until there is either a cure for diabetes or an affordable, reliable, internal artificial pancreas, an insulin pump is the next best thing. Characteristics of a person who would do well pumping insulin include someone

1. on intensive insulin therapy (three or more injections per day) but not meeting glycemic goals,
2. able and willing to make appropriate insulin adjustments based on frequent blood sugar testing,
3. well motivated to learn pump technology and able to follow through and make the necessary changes,
4. desirous of or requiring a more flexible lifestyle with regard to meals and exercise,
5. willing to be tethered via tubing to a small box housing a continuous flow of rapid-acting insulin,
6. with added incentive to control blood sugar prior to and during pregnancy,
7. having adequate health insurance to help with cost, and, perhaps most importantly,
8. with a take-charge personality willing to do whatever it takes to make it work.

Pumping insulin is definitely worth the hassles involved. When I was put on my first insulin pump after working at blood sugar control for 10 years with 4 to 5 injections a day, I felt like I finally had my life back. I could eat and exercise when I wanted without worrying about when my intermediate-acting insulin was going to peak. When the insulin analogs became available, insulin decision making became even easier. I could eat what I wanted when I wanted, within reason, just like anyone else. However, monitoring blood sugars to set basal rates throughout the day and night meant pre- and postmeal testing, as well as testing two or three times during the night. Pumping insulin is not the answer for everyone. It takes effort, willingness to experiment, and the ability to follow through to use an insulin pump successfully. Blood sugars usually level out so that the roller coaster ride of highs and lows, often in the same day, rarely occurs. Blood sugars are more predictable, and food, physical activity, and insulin doses finally make sense.

Deciding to go on an insulin pump does have its aggravations. Pump alarms for low volume, low battery, and "no delivery" are important safety precautions but can be annoying. However, they can usually be set to vibrate. The "no delivery" alarm must be tended to very quickly because very high blood sugars and diabetic ketoacidosis can ensue in a matter of hours. Most pumpers use rapid-acting insulin analogs in their pumps, which have a very short duration of action (see Table 4.2). Tubing, reservoirs, and insulin must be readily available at work and at home, as well as anywhere the client might be, for this potential emergency. A low battery is less problematic because most pumps will continue to function for 8 or more hours. A pump rarely malfunctions, but the 1-800 number on the back of the pump is manned 24/7 to help a person troubleshoot problems and reprogram the pump. It is probably wise to keep an up-to-date written record of all basal rates so they can be reset. If there is a delay in fixing any glitch, syringes and insulin must be available as backup. That brings us to the "stuff" that pump users need to carry with them. Anyone diagnosed with type 1 or type 2 diabetes should carry medication that must be taken with meals as well as a glucose monitor, strips, a lancing device and lancets, tissues, a log book, and spare batteries for the monitor. Most monitors come with convenient carrying cases for that purpose. Additionally, anyone on insulin should have available unexpired insulin, syringes, and alcohol swabs. Pumpers also need extra reservoirs and tubing, fresh pump batteries, and any other paraphernalia needed to change insulin setup and/or insertion site. There are coolers, pouches, and carrying cases for this purpose. Supplies can also be carried in a purse, backpack, fanny pack, or briefcase. If not refrigerated, insulin at room temperature will maintain its potency for at least 1 month. Do not, however, freeze or leave insulin in 90-degree weather—leaving it in the glove compartment of a car, even in spring or fall, is a bad idea.

Most people who use insulin pumps use the abdomen as their insertion site, upper abdomen for men and lower abdomen for women. However, all appropriate subcutaneous sites for insulin injection, such as the anterior thigh, back of the upper arm, and upper buttocks, can be used. The insertion site should be changed every 2–3 days to prevent irritation and infection. Pumps can be removed for bathing, swimming, contact sports, and sexual activity for up to 2 hours if blood sugars are well controlled. When reconnected, a blood sugar should be taken, and an appropriate bolus dose, if needed, should be given.

Persons using insulin pumps need a support system, both professionally and personally. A supportive diabetes educator and/or endocrinologist can help to troubleshoot any pump and/or blood sugar difficulties. Selected family members, friends, and/or coworkers should be informed as to how they can help in meaningful ways. This may mean that they demonstrate their concern by asking about blood sugars/meal preferences, providing privacy, a regular Coke, or other fast-acting sugar source when hypoglycemia is a problem, or none of the above except when asked. Wearing an insulin pump is a serious financial and personal commitment to controlling blood sugars and managing diabetes while decreasing hypoglycemic episodes and increasing lifestyle flexibility. Insulin pumps are not just appropriate for type 1 diabetics but for type 2 as well. Children as young as 1 year old can also be managed well with an insulin pump (Fox, Buckloh, Smith, Wysocki, & Mauras, 2005). Parents can set lock-out controls so that young children can not change settings. (See chapter 8 for more discussion about children and diabetes.)

Other Injectable Diabetes Medication

Two new subcutaneous injectable medications have been recently added to the arsenal of drugs to control blood sugar. The first is pramlintide (Symlin), a synthetic amylin hormone that is normally produced by the beta cells of the pancreas as is insulin. Pramlintide injections given with meals that contain at least 250 calories and 30 grams of carbohydrate should not cause hypoglycemia or weight gain, as insulin does, and may even promote weight loss. It should be given with rapid-acting insulin at meals but cannot be mixed in the same syringe, and the amount of rapid-acting insulin given before a meal should be lowered by 50%. Symlin is dosed in micrograms (µg or mcg) with a conversion chart to units so patients can use insulin syringes. However, this may cause confusion on the part of clients and their families and prescribers and dispensers of the drug such as pharmacists and nurses who are unfamiliar with the medication and the conversion chart. (See Table 4.3 for this conversion.) This table should be posted in all nursing stations or wherever medications are prepared to insure that the proper dose is administered. Because some of the unit doses are measured in half units, only low-dose (50-unit) or 30-unit syringes should be used, as there is more space between each unit to allow for better accuracy. Symlin must be refrigerated, except for open vials, which are good for 28 days at room temperature. Avoid freezing or exposure to a temperature above 77°F.

TABLE 4.3 Conversion Table for Doses of Symlin (Pramlintide) for Subcutaneous Injection

Dose in micrograms (µg or mcg)	Draw up this amount in U-100 insulin syringe (units)
15 mcg	2.5 Units
30 mcg	5.0 Units
45 mcg	7.5 Units
60 mcg	10.0 Units
120 mcg	20.0 Units

Note. Adapted from Symlin Medication Guide, http://www.symlin.com/pdf/SYMLIN-Ann-PI.pdf, Amylin Pharmaceuticals, Inc.

Symlin slows stomach emptying and decreases postprandial elevations of blood glucose. Patients are advised to test blood sugar before meals, 2 hours after meals, and at bedtime. Obviously, this drug is not for everyone. Symlin has been approved for use with type 1 and type 2 diabetics using rapid-onset or regular insulin as a premeal bolus dose and who are not achieving glycemic control on their present regimen and are well motivated to follow directions carefully. The most common side effect is nausea, which improves after a few weeks. The dose is started low and is titrated up until the desired effect is achieved.

Symlin   Amylin Pharmaceuticals, Inc.   http://www.symlin.com

The second new injectable drug developed for use in treating diabetes is exenatide (Byetta), which is the first in a new class of medications for type 2 diabetes called incretin mimetics. It is a synthetic version of the human incretin hormone GLP-1 (glucagon-like peptide-1) that is secreted in the small intestines, but it has a longer half-life. Byetta helps the body to self-regulate glycemic control. It enhances insulin secretion only when blood sugar is elevated and decreases insulin production as blood sugar normalizes (Clark, 2006). According to its manufacturer, this drug is indicated for clients with type 2 diabetes who are taking metformin or a sulfonylurea or both without achieving glycemic control. Byetta is used in conjunction with these medications, although the dose of metformin and/ or sulfonylurea may need to be reduced. Byetta is dispensed in prefilled 30-day supply pens of 5 mcg or 10 mcg, depending on which dose is prescribed. It is given twice a day as a subcutaneous injection within 60 minutes of eating breakfast and dinner.

GLP-1 hormone is structurally similar to glucagon but acts very differently. Whereas glucagon from the alpha cells of the pancreas causes the release of stored glucose from the liver to prevent hypoglycemia, GLP-1 enhances insulin secretion but only when glucose is elevated, for example, after meals. It also

1. suppresses inappropriate glucagon secretion (a problem in type 2 diabetes),
2. promotes satiety, which may decrease food intake, and
3. slows gastric emptying, thus decreasing the spike of postprandial blood sugar (another problem in type 2 diabetes).

The most common side effect is nausea, which decreases over time. Byetta pens should be stored in the original carton (protected from the light) and in the refrigerator. Once in use, the pen should be refrigerated or kept cold but never frozen. After 30 days, the pen should be thrown away even if it still contains medication. The pen needles should be attached right before use and properly discarded after use. Leaving needles on the pen may cause leaking or air bubbles.

Byetta	Amylin Pharmaceuticals, Inc. & Eli Lilly Company	http://www.byetta.com

INHALED INSULIN

One of the most anticipated alternatives to injected insulin has finally arrived. Since insulin was discovered in the 1920s, scientists have been working to try to develop an inhaled form of insulin. For the last 15 years or so, there has been more intense interest in insulin delivery alternatives since the technology now exists to finally make them a reality. Nasal insulin, oral insulin, buccal administered gels, and insulin patches, as well as inhaled insulin, have been studied. Exubera, a form of powdered, fast-acting, inhaled human insulin, developed by Pfizer Inc. using a pulmonary inhaler manufactured by Nektar Therapeutics, was approved by both the European Medicine Agency (EMA) and the U.S. Food and Drug Administration (FDA) in February 2006 and has been available in Europe since June 2006.

Preprandial Exubera and twice-daily NPH insulin have been tested in type 1 diabetics (ages 12–65) and have been shown to be comparable to premeal injections of regular insulin and twice-daily NPH insulin (Skyler et al., 2005). Phase III trials using preprandial Exubera alone or in conjunction with oral hypoglycemic agents (sulfonylureas, metformin, or insulin sensitizers such as Actos or Avandia) have demonstrated superior glucose control in type 2 diabetics on oral hypoglycemics not achieving acceptable hemoglobin A_{1c} (Rosenstock et al., 2005). The most exciting news is the improvement in patient satisfaction in both Exubera-treated groups. Clients with type 2 diabetes either continued their oral hypoglycemic medication and added one or two inhalations of Exubera prior to eating or simply used the premeal Exubera alone to lower their hemoglobin A_{1c} (Rosenstock et al., 2005). In a 12-week, randomized, comparative trial with type 2 diabetics not controlled with diet and exercise, DeFronzo et al. (2005) reported improved glycemic control with inhaled human insulin compared to rosiglitazone (Avandia). Avandia is a first-line drug in the treatment of type 2 diabetes not controlled by diet and exercise. This study suggests that inhaled human insulin is more effective in controlling blood sugar than a first-line drug and could be used early in the treatment of type 2 diabetes (DeFronzo et al., 2005) In another 6-month study, it was reported that Exubera "appears to be effective, well tolerated, and well accepted in patients with type 2 diabetes and provides glycemic control comparable to a conventional subcutaneous regimen" (Hollander et al., 2004, p. 2356). With the availability of newer long-acting insulins like Lantus, it is now possible for insulin-using type 1 and type 2 diabetics to be treated with premeal Exubera and just one injection per day of a basal insulin.

The most important potential gain from the use of inhaled insulin is that physicians reluctant to put their type 2 patients on injectable insulin (Peyrot, 2005) for improved glycemic control may now do so. Clients reluctant to comply with the need for insulin may now embrace the noninjectable method of delivery. It is estimated that 40% of type 2 diabetics already need insulin to achieve good control of blood glucose (Saudek & Margolis, 2006). Because type 2 diabetes is progressive, most clients who live long enough with the disease will need insulin for glycemic control. The bottom line in preventing long-term complications is normalizing blood sugars. Now that an acceptable delivery option for insulin is available, there is the potential that many long-term complications could be prevented or delayed in the type 2 diabetes population.

Exubera comes in 1 mg and 3 mg powder blister packs that are aerosolized by a pulmonary inhaler and absorbed into the alveolar capillary bloodstream. Odegard and Capoccia state, "Dry powder formulations can deliver a higher dose per puff, are stable at room temperature, and can resist microbial growth compared to liquid formulations" (Odegard & Capoccia, 2005, p. 845). The conversion to units is roughly 2–3 units per mg. However, the recommended starting dose is 0.15 mg per kilogram of body weight divided into three approximately equal premeal doses. The onset of action of Exubera is more rapid than injected regular insulin but lasts as long, thus controlling postprandial glucose spikes common in type 2 diabetes. Exubera's onset of action is 31 minutes versus 54 minutes with regular insulin. Its peak action is 108 minutes versus 147 minutes with regular insulin, and its duration of action is approximately 6 hours, comparable to regular insulin. "Despite a similar duration of action, inhaled insulin has demonstrated lower rates of hypoglycemia than subcutaneous regular insulin" (Odegard & Capoccia, 2005, p. 845).

Exubera is currently only approved for type 1 and type 2 adult clients and is contraindicated for smokers because smoking causes faster absorption. It is not recommended at this time for clients with asthma, bronchitis, or emphysema. The most common side effect is coughing, which subsides with use. Baseline lung function studies should be done at the beginning of treatment and repeated every 6 to 12 months (ADA, 2006).

Most type 1 clients on inhaled human insulin experienced a mild weight gain that was less than the injectable insulin group (Quattrin, Bélanger, Bohannon, & Schwartz, 2004), and type 2 diabetics experienced much less weight gain with Exubera versus injectable insulin (Hollander et al., 2004).

So if you or a client has been "waiting to inhale," the wait is over.

The explosion of new types of insulin and oral and injectable medication to treat the ever-increasing number of people diagnosed with diabetes should continue to proliferate in the years to come. Nurses must keep themselves updated by attending workshops and/or subscribing to nursing journals or free online listservs like Medscape (http://www. medscape.com) if they are to give competent and effective care to clients with diabetes. Again, research on new drugs can be accessed on the Web by Googling (http://www.google.com) the drug trade names or going to the manufacturers' Web sites.

REFERENCES

American Diabetes Association. (2003). *Insulin therapy in the 21st century.* Alexandria, VA: Author.

American Diabetes Association. (2006, April). Inhalable insulin is on the way. *Diabetes Forecast,* p. 15.

Clark, W. L. (2006, January-February). Exenatide: From the Gila monster to you. *Diabetes Self-Management,* pp. 36–40.

DeFronzo, R., Bergenstal, R. M., Cefalu, W. T., Pullman, J., Lerman, S., Bode, B. W., et al. (2005, August). Efficacy of inhaled insulin in patients with type 2 diabetes not controlled with diet and exercise. *Diabetes Care, 28,* 1922–1928.

Fox, L. A., Buckloh, L. M., Smith, S. D., Wysocki, T., & Mauras, N. (2005). A randomized controlled trial of insulin pump therapy in young children with type 1 diabetes. *Diabetes Care, 28,* 1277–1281.

Hollander, P., Blonde, L., Rowe, R., Mehta, A. E., Milburn, J. L., Hershon, K. S., et al. (2004, October). Efficacy and safety of inhaled insulin (Exubera) compared with subcutaneous insulin therapy in patients with type 2 diabetes. *Diabetes Care, 27,* 2356–2362.

Odegard, P. S., & Capoccia, K. L. (2005, May). Inhaled insulin: Exubera. *The Annals of Pharmacotherapy, 39,* 843–853.

Peyrot, M. (2005, November). Resistance to insulin therapy among patients and providers. *Diabetes Care, 28,* 2673–2679.

Quattrin, T., Bélanger, A., Bohannon, N. J. V., Schwartz, S. L. (2004, November). Efficacy and safety of inhaled insulin (Exubera) compared with subcutaneous insulin therapy in patients with type 1 diabetes. *Diabetes Care, 27,* 2622–2627.

Rosenstock, J., Zinman, B., Murphy, L. J., Clement, S. C., Moore, P., Bowering, C. K., et al. (2005). Inhaled insulin improves glycemic control when substituted for or added to oral combinations therapy in type 2 diabetes. *Annals of Internal Medicine, 143,* 549–558.

Saudek, C. D., & Margolis, S. (2006). *Johns Hopkins white papers: Diabetes.* Redding, CT: Medletter Associates.

Skyler, J. S., Weinstock, R. S., Raskin, P., Yale, J.-F., Barrett, E., Gerich, J. E., et al. (2005, July). Use of inhaled insulin in a basal/bolus insulin regimen in type 1 diabetic subjects. *Diabetes Care, 28,* 1630–1635.

5

Glycemic Control

Control will set you free.

Anonymous

The bottom line with diabetes treatment is attaining near-normal blood sugars while minimizing hypoglycemic episodes. Several research studies, including the Diabetes Control and Complications Trial (DCCT) with type 1 diabetics and the United Kingdom Prospective Diabetes Study (UKPDS) with type 2 diabetics, have shown significant prevention or delay of chronic complications related to hyperglycemia as a result of tight control of blood sugars (ADA, 2003).

Currently, the American Diabetes Association (2006, p. S60) recommends the following goals for blood sugar control for type 1 and type 2 diabetes:

Fasting	70–99 mg/dl
Before meals	90–130 mg/dl
Peak 1–2 hours after meal	< 180 mg/dl
Hemoglobin A_{1c}	< 7.0%

Nondiabetics have a hemoglobin A_{1c} of 4.0%–6.0%. A1C is a measurement of the percentage of glycosylation (how sugared) the average hemoglobin molecule experiences over a period of 2–3 months floating in blood containing glucose. Glucose of varying amounts is present in the blood and "sticks" to hemoglobin. The red cells, which contain the hemoglobin, live for about 120 days, so the glycosylated hemoglobin of these red cells represents an average blood glucose level during this time period. As you can see in Table 5.1, the higher the A1C, the higher the average blood glucose. Therefore, following nutritional recommendations the week before an office visit really does not affect the results. The American Diabetes Association also recommends that glycemic goals be individualized, especially with children, the elderly, and clients who are pregnant or who have frequent and severe hypoglycemia (ADA, 2006). Glucose readings after meals may be particularly difficult to control in clients not on insulin therapy, thus causing a higher A1C average. Additionally, frequent low blood sugars may cancel out high blood sugars, thus lowering the A1C average and creating an artificially appropriate-looking percentage. This is an important point to remember. For example, prior to using an insulin pump, my A1Cs were usually between 5% and 6%. However, I had frequent high and low blood sugars and my lows, especially during the night, were more significant. My seemingly great glycemic control actually indicated that I rode the blood sugar roller coaster most of the time. Since I have been using an insulin pump, my hypoglycemic episodes are very infrequent and any high blood sugars are more noticeable. Thus, my A1Cs, usually between 6.5% and 7%, are a truer reflection of my glycemic control.

Normal fasting blood sugar was decreased by the American Diabetes Association from the 1997 guidelines of 70 to 110 mg/dl to 70 to 99 mg/dl in 2003. This increased the span for impaired glucose tolerance from 110 to 125 mg/dl to 100 to 125 mg/dl, which is now called prediabetes. The purpose of both changes is to alert more patients and their health

TABLE 5.1 Correlation Between A1C Level and Mean Plasma Glucose Levels on Multiple Testing Over 2–3 Months

A1C (%)	Mean plasma glucose	
	mg/dl	mmol/l
6	135	7.5
7	170	9.5
8	205	11.5
9	240	13.5
10	275	15.5
11	310	17.5
12	345	19.5

Note. From "Standards of Medical Care in Diabetes—2006," by the American Diabetes Association, 2006, Diabetes Care, 29, S4–S42. Copyright © 2006 by the American Diabetes Association. Reprinted with permission from the American Diabetes Association.

care providers to the potential damage that can occur prior to the official diagnosis of diabetes at a blood sugar of 126 mg/dl. The hope is that this will be a wake-up call for lifestyle modifications and weight loss, if needed, which should prevent or delay the onset of type 2 diabetes. Individualizing our approach to clients is covered in depth in part 2 of this book.

HYPERGLYCEMIA

Technically, higher than normal blood sugar is defined as anything above the levels given at the beginning of this chapter. The glucose levels depend on the timing of food intake from fasting and preprandial levels to 1–2 hours postprandial levels. Most people with diabetes have no symptoms until blood sugar approaches 250 mg/dl. This is an important point to make with clients who do not routinely monitor their glucose levels. The most common symptoms include frequent urination of very dilute urine, thirst from the loss of body fluids in the urine, and hunger for simple sugars. Other symptoms may include the following:

- headache, sleepiness, difficulty concentrating
- visual disturbances from the glucose concentration in the eye fluids
- dry or flushed skin from dehydration
- general malaise

These symptoms may be so common that older clients may think they are a normal part of aging. When illness, even the common cold, or other stressors increase blood sugars to 400 mg/dl and higher, ketoacidosis can occur. When the body does not have enough insulin to move glucose into cells for energy, the cells turn to fat to provide needed fuel. The metabolism of fat produces fatty acids and ketones that accumulate in the blood and affect the brain, producing the symptoms listed above. The kidneys try to eliminate ketones and glucose, giving rise to ketonuria and glucosuria. Testing urine for ketones is confirmation that ketoacidosis is occurring. Other symptoms of this very dangerous condition include the following:

- shortness of breath
- fruity smelling breath (more like the acetone of nail polish remover)
- nausea and vomiting

If ketoacidosis persists, the client will lapse into a coma. The blood sugar level that produces a coma is very individualized and can be anywhere from 600 mg/dl to 1,500 mg/dl or higher. This condition occurs mostly with type 1 diabetes and is caused by omitting an insulin dose, eating excessive amounts of carbohydrates, illness, and some medications (see Table 5.2). However, these same conditions, if severe enough, can overwhelm the ability of the pancreas of a type 2 diabetic to respond to oral agents by increasing production of insulin. When this happens, the type 2 diabetic can become ketotic. Do not assume that just because someone has type 2 diabetes, he or she cannot develop ketoacidosis. On the other hand, when ketones are *not* present in the unconscious type 2 diabetic, the resulting condition is called hyperosmolar nonketosis. This may happen in an older client who lapses into a coma from the severe dehydration caused by hyperglycemia. What all diabetics need to realize is that paying attention to blood sugars may become a life or death decision.

Factors That Raise Blood Sugar

Table 5.2 lists the many factors that affect blood sugar by decreasing the effectiveness of insulin or by increasing the need for insulin to control blood sugar. Most nurses are aware that physical stress, such as a heart attack, a stroke, trauma, pain, surgery, or infection, increases blood sugar by increasing stress hormones such as epinephrine and norepinephrine. This reaction represents the old fight-or-flight instinct we inherited from our prehistoric ancestors. We no longer have to fight the saber-toothed tiger or flee from the woolly mammoth, but our adrenal glands secrete adrenalin anyway.

What we need in order to fight or flee is sufficient blood pressure (arteries vasoconstrict), increased cardiac output (heart rate increases), sufficient oxygen to hook on to each red cell being pumped out (respiratory rate increases and bronchioles dilate), *and* extra glucose to fuel our brain to think and our muscles to move. Under the influence of stress hormones, stored glucose is dumped into the bloodstream by the liver and skeletal muscles. During times of physical stress, all diabetics need more insulin even if they are not eating (NPO). Type 2 diabetics who use oral medication to control blood sugars may need rapid-acting insulin during the stressful

TABLE 5.2 Factors That Affect Blood Sugar

Factors that increase blood sugar	Factors that decrease blood sugar
Skipping antidiabetic medication	**Too much antidiabetic medication**
Overeating, especially carbohydrates	**Skipping a meal after taking medication**
Significant weight gain	**Significant weight loss**
Decreased physical activity	**Increased physical activity** even several hours later
Medication Corticosteroids Thyroid supplements Diuretics Caffeine (high doses) Niacin (high doses)	**Medications** Beta blockers MAO inhibitors Nicotine patch Ritalin
Hormones Stress hormones (adrenaline) Growth hormones Cortisol Pregnancy hormones (2nd & 3rd trimesters) Hormones during menses Estrogen	**Pregnancy** (1st trimester) **Stress management** **Alcohol** **Other** Heat and humidity High altitude Intense brain activity New or unusual surroundings Socializing Stimulating environment
Emotions Anger Depression Fear Panic	
Other Excessive sleeping	

crisis. However, if the insulin sliding scale starts at 200 mg/dl, we need to advocate for our clients to get that lowered to at least 150 mg/dl. Even critically ill patients should maintain blood sugar less than 180 mg/dl (ADA, 2006, p. S29).

Inadequate glycemic control during hospitalization puts patients at risk for infection and poor wound healing (ADA, 2006, p. S29). The fear of hypoglycemia is what drives these inadequate sliding scales. Testing blood sugars every 4 hours would demonstrate that hypoglycemia does not occur in an insulin-resistant type 2 diabetic who becomes even more insulin-resistant with stress hormones. The same hormonal reaction occurs, of course, with the psychological stressors of fear, anxiety, depression, anger, and so forth. These reactions to hospitalization only add to the increase of blood sugar from physical stress. Nurses may be able to decrease some of the psychological stressors by being good listeners, providing prompt and adequate pain control, and explaining all procedures on the client's level, thus developing a trusting therapeutic relationship.

There are several medications that also increase cellular insulin resistance or that antagonize the action of insulin. The most common is prednisone or any corticosteroid given to control the inflammatory process. Clients dealing with severe asthma, rheumatoid arthritis, systemic lupus erythematosis (SLE), as well as dermotologic, hematologic, and neurologic conditions may be treated with a corticosteroid. Even a corticosteroid injected into the spine or a painful joint or given as eye drops can elevate blood sugar in a person with diabetes. Other problematic hormones that can raise blood sugar include thyroxin, growth hormone, estrogen as part of the menstrual cycle or taken after menopause, and several placental hormones that increase in the second half of pregnancy. Any person not able to increase production of insulin to counter these insulin antagonists will develop hyperglycemia. Other drugs that may increase the need for insulin include some diuretics like hydrochlorothiazide (HCTZ), Lasix, and Bumex, and large doses of caffeine. In addition, weight gain itself increases insulin resistance, as does excessive sleep (Scheiner, 2004).

HYPOGLYCEMIA

Anyone with diabetes, especially clients taking insulin or oral hypoglycemic agents, can experience low blood sugar. If the intake of carbohydrates does not match the amount of insulin injected or produced by the pancreas as a result of an oral sulfonylurea, blood sugar will drop. Everyone has his or her own reaction to hypoglycemia. However, most have the following symptoms:

- tremors, shakiness, or jerky movements
- sweating, pale moist skin
- dizziness, feeling faint, headache
- excessive hunger, especially for carbohydrates

- sudden, atypical change in behavior, mood swings, or erratic behavior
- tingling or numbness around the mouth or tongue
- difficulty paying attention, confusion
- visual disturbances, difficulty reading, dilated pupils
- increased heart and respiratory rates
- seizures and coma

As you can see, some of these symptoms sound very similar to those of hyperglycemia. It is important for diabetics to confirm these symptoms with glucose monitoring so that the meaning is clear. Because the need to treat a low blood sugar is fairly immediate to prevent brain cell damage, clients should be taught that when in doubt, eat. Sometimes the client may realize that he or she has administered insulin and not eaten or exercised before eating and will know that the symptoms are probably related to hypoglycemia.

Treatments for low blood sugar include a 1/2 cup of unsweetened orange juice, 5–6 hard candies (not sugar-free), 3–4 glucose tablets, or a packet of glucose gel. The last two items can be found over the counter in most drugstores and should be carried by anyone prone to hypoglycemia, including anyone on insulin, regardless of whether they have type 1 or type 2 diabetes.

Factors That Decrease Blood Sugar

Chapter 3 provides an explanation of how increased physical activity, including sexual activity, improves cellular insulin sensitivity and decreases insulin needs, perhaps for hours. If the amount of insulin injected is not decreased or more carbohydrates are not ingested, hypoglycemia may result. In the same fashion, the amount of carbohydrates, both simple and complex, must match the amount of insulin secreted by the pancreas or given by injection or pump. With the advent of rapid-acting insulin analogs, clients can wait until a meal is served to decide how many carbs (see "Carb Counting" in chapter 2) they plan to ingest and then deliver an appropriate amount of insulin. If a client is taking a rapid-acting secretagogue such as Prandin or Starlix with each meal, he or she can omit taking it if skipping a meal or if no or very few carbohydrate foods are consumed. The problem of needing to eat carbohydrate foods occurs when a client has injected intermediate-acting insulin (NPH or lente) in the morning, which will peak around lunch time, or has taken a long-acting secretagogue (any of the sulfonylureas) with breakfast, which will increase the amount of insulin secreted all day long. If the carbs do not match the insulin, low blood sugar will result. In the above circumstances, the client must eat meals on time and provide a similar amount of carbohydrates at each of these meals.

Drugs that often decrease blood sugar include beta-blockers for hypertension or arrhythmias, MAO inhibitors for depression, nicotine patches, and Ritalin. A good medication history may unearth the cause of unexpected hypoglycemia. Alcohol also lowers blood sugar and should always be consumed with food. If a significant drop in blood sugar occurs after ingesting alcohol, the liver may not be able to respond to glucagon secreted by the alpha cells of the pancreas, resulting in no stored glucose being released. This can be a potentially dangerous situation. Other factors that can potentially lower blood sugar include excessive heat and humidity (especially while exercising), high altitudes, and anything that may distract you from your usual routine of checking blood sugar, such as socializing, new or unusual surroundings, a stimulating environment, or intense brain work (Scheiner, 2004). During these times it is important to monitor blood sugars periodically and often. Table 5.2 summarizes factors that decrease blood glucose.

Hypoglycemia Unawareness

Some type 1 diabetics may no longer sense an impending low blood sugar and may simply become unconscious when blood sugars are low enough. Because brain cells only burn glucose for energy, they stop functioning and may even die when blood glucose plummets. This very dangerous condition may affect people with long-standing type 1 diabetes, those who have neuropathy preventing the occurrence of symptoms, those who experience frequent low blood sugars (several time a week) as a result of tight glucose control, or those who are on beta-blockers for cardiac arrhythmias or hypertension. Beta-blockers blunt the effects of epinephrine and norepinephrine in response to a low blood sugar. Some people begin to have different symptoms as the years go by and simply fail to acknowledge them as a signal to eat something and raise blood sugars. In either case, frequent blood sugar monitoring is crucial, and eating multiple small meals is a necessity. Alerting others that a client lives with or works with is essential. Having a Glucagon kit and teaching others to administer the injection may become a life-saving measure. The dosage depends on the age of the client:

Infants to 3 years old	1/4 mg or 0.25 mL
4 to 11 years old	1/2 mg or 0.5 mL
12 years old to adult	1 mg or 1 mL

A good video by the American Diabetes Association on how to administer the hormone can be viewed at http://www.diabetes.org/type-1-diabetes/hypoglycemia.jsp.

BLOOD GLUCOSE MONITORING

There are many blood glucose meters on the market that rely on electrophoresis to read blood sugar. Most require a drop of blood from the finger; however, alternative sites, such as the forearm or the area of the palm below the thumb, may be used with certain types of meters. The area tested should be washed with warm water and soap to provide a surface free of debris or food residue and to increase the blood supply to the area. To increase the size of the drop of blood, massage the area, let the arm hang down, and/or milk the finger. To ensure accuracy, follow the manufacturer's direction as to coding the meter with each package of strips. Strips must be protected from heat and humidity. Periodic testing of strips and meter with the appropriate control solution is necessary, especially if the glucose reading is in question. When in doubt, throw the package of strips out. If a new package does not solve the problem, call the help-line number on the back of the meter. Most companies will help to troubleshoot problems and/or send a replacement meter. There are lancing devices and lancets to fit every client's coordination need and depth of skin, so clients should be encouraged to experiment with others if the one that came with the meter is not satisfactory. Meters today require a very small drop of blood. The resource guide provided by the American Diabetes Association at http://www.diabetes.org/diabetes-forecast/resource-guide.jsp provides information and comparisons for meters, strips, lancing devices, lancets, syringes, and many other supplies. Another good source to help evaluate the particulars of meters, including A1C meters and kits, is http://www.mendosa.com/meters.htm.

Frequent blood sugar monitoring is recommended for both type 1 and type 2 clients. I am frequently asked how often to test and my answer is "whenever you need the information." (See Table 5.3 for guidelines.) Today with all of the devices available, it is inconceivable to me that anyone would persist in wondering what their blood sugar is. If a person feels bad or odd, it is a simple procedure to rule in or rule out blood sugar as a cause. For a long time, insurance companies did not cover glucose strips (the expensive part of following blood sugars) for type 2 diabetics unless they were on insulin—sort of a penny-wise and pound-foolish approach. Today, several states have passed laws that mandate that insurance companies cover meters, strips, lancing devices, and lancets, as well as diabetes education for anyone diagnosed. Many physicians still do not ask their type 2 patients to test blood sugars, or if they do, the testing is very sporadic. In order to understand how food and physical activity affects each individual, that person must test his or her blood sugar. Doing lab work only at a doctor's office visit is really too little, too late. Living with blood sugars in the 200s or higher is causing tissue damage. The sooner hyperglycemia is discovered and treated, the less damage is done.

What should a client do with the glucose monitor numbers? Currently there are many options from low-tech lifestyle changes like omitting or

TABLE 5.3 Rules to Follow for Glycemic Control

1.	Carry blood glucose meter and supplies at all times.
2.	Test blood sugar often, especially before eating, taking diabetes medication that will increase the amount of insulin in the blood, going to bed, or experiencing physical or emotional stress including physical activity.
3.	If using intermediate-acting insulin (NPH) or a long-acting secretagogue, eat on a preset schedule with a predetermined amount of carbohydrates.
4.	Take rapid-acting insulin or short-acting secretagogue only immediately before eating a meal with carbohydrates.
5.	If hypoglycemia is a potential problem, always carry fast-acting glucose such as gels or tablets available at drugstores.
6.	Always carry extra supplies needed to correct potential high blood sugar, such as extra insulin and syringes even if using an insulin pump and other antidiabetic medication if prescribed.
7.	Check expiration dates and protect supplies from extremes of heat and cold.

decreasing the amount of certain foods or increasing physical activity to changing medication regimens to include administration of insulin via syringe, pump, or inhaler. Checking a blood sugar 1–2 hours after eating pizza or taking a 30-minute walk is more convincing to a client than anything he or she can read or hear from a health care provider. The increased blood sugar from eating excessive amounts of carbohydrates or the normalizing of blood sugar provided by simple exercise is very empowering.

Most people are not convinced to change their lifestyle with scare tactics warning of the development of chronic complications in 20 years' time. The convincing evidence needs to be more immediate. Glycemic control improves personal well-being right now. It prevents infections and improves health. As a client redefines his or her goals in life based on improved glycemic control and his or her health in general, he or she will be encouraged to continue to eat nutritiously, lose weight, increase physical activity, and follow the resulting blood sugars and periodic A1C percentages. Clients and health care practitioners alike must also remember that no one is perfect. Blood glucose numbers are neither good nor bad. They are simply data that help us to make better choices now and in the future.

Continuous Blood Glucose Monitors

Medtronic-MiniMed, one of the companies that manufacture insulin pumps, has developed a continuous glucose monitoring system. It provides 3 days' worth of glucose level information when data are downloaded to a computer using the accompanying software. The sensor measures glucose levels in the interstitial fluid every 10 seconds and averages these every 5 minutes. The data is printed in a graphic presentation. Rather than taking glucose readings 3–6 times per day, this data are continuous, so what happens between readings is clearly shown.

A glucose sensor is inserted into the subcutaneous tissue much like inserting the catheter for an insulin pump. This sensor measures glucose in the interstitial fluid and sends this information to an external glucose monitor that compiles and stores 72 hours of data. The person wearing the sensor must enter at least three blood glucose readings from a standard glucose meter as well as insulin dosages, exercise, and content of meals. At the end of 3 days, the information is downloaded at the physician's office and appropriate adjustment in insulin regimen and the timing of exercise and meals can be made.

Medtronic-MiniMed has also developed the Guardian RT Continuous Glucose Monitoring System, which has recently been approved by the FDA for clients over 18 years old with either type 1 or type 2 diabetes. The Guardian RT system is a continuous glucose monitoring system that displays current blood sugar every 5 minutes. It is programmed to alert the patients when glucose levels register preset values that are too high or too low. This information will help patients take action to avoid both hyperglycemic and hypoglycemic episodes. A transmitter connected to the glucose sensor is attached to the skin by an adhesive patch. Using a radio frequency, it sends glucose values to the monitor every 5 minutes. The monitor displays glucose values and sounds an alarm or vibrates if values are too high or low. The sensor and transmitter are waterproof, but the monitor is not; however, it can receive signals from the transmitter up to 6 feet away. Using special software, the monitor information can be downloaded to a computer and viewed or printed as graphs, charts, and tables. This technology is only available in a few cities at the present time. Studies have shown that continuous glucose monitoring motivates clients to improve self-management, thus reducing their hemoglobin A_{1c}. Reduction in the A1C percentage reduces the risk of microvascular and neuropathic long-term complications (ADA, 2006, p. S9). More information on the Guardian RT can be found at http://www.minimed. com/products/guardianrt/index.html.

DexCom is another company working on continuous glucose monitoring sensors. The DexCom STS Continuous Monitoring System is a short-term sensor that transmits blood glucose values wirelessly to the DexCom STS Hand Held Receiver. This device is inserted just under the skin by the patient, held in place on the skin with adhesive, and worn for up to 3 days. DexCom received approval with the U.S. Food and Drug Administration in March 2006. DexCom also has developed a long-term continuous glucose sensor that is inserted in the abdomen by a physician in a short outpatient procedure under a local anesthetic. It is designed to function in the same manner as the short-term sensor but for 1 year. Then it is removed by a physician and another is inserted. The outcome data for clinical trials for both sensors demonstrate significant improvement in glucose profiles when clients have access to continuous glucose monitoring to help them manage their disease (Garg, Schwartz, & Edelman, 2004). More information about DexCom's continuous monitoring systems can be found at http://www. dexcom.com.

The GlucoWatch G2 Biographer is worn like a wristwatch. It uses imperceptible electric currents to draw interstitial fluid through the skin into gel pads in the device, which then measures the glucose in this fluid. The Biographer compares each 10-minute reading with a high and low setting selected. An alarm is sounded if glucose readings are at these settings or trending toward the low alert. This device requires a prescription, stores readings for up to 13 hours at a time, detects trends, and tracks patterns of glucose levels over time. It is designed to be used in conjunction with a regular blood glucose meter (http://www.glucowatch.com).

The most important value of any glucose monitoring device is its impact on diabetes management. Obviously the more data a client has, the more he or she can analyze the information and make frequent corrections, which should result in greater glucose control, lower A1C percentage, and prevention of both acute and chronic complications. The better the blood sugar control, the more options a client has and the more normal and fulfilling life can be. Control of blood sugars by whatever means necessary and available can leave a person free to enjoy life to the fullest. That should be the goal and the mantra of all diabetics as well as the nurses and practitioners who serve them.

REFERENCES

American Diabetes Association. (2003). *Insulin therapy in the 21st century.* Alexandria, VA: Author.
American Diabetes Association. (2006). Diabetes management in correctional institutions. *Diabetes Care, 29,* S59–S66.
Garg, S., Schwartz, S., & Edelman, S. (2004). Improved glucose excursions using an implantable real-time continuous glucose sensor in adults with type 1 diabetes. *Diabetes Care, 27,* 734–738.
Scheiner, G. (2004). *Think like a pancreas.* New York: Marlowe & Company.

6

The Cure Is Near

When one door of happiness closes, another opens; but often we look so long at the closed door that we do not see the one which has opened for us.

Helen Keller

The goal of the American Diabetes Association (ADA) and the Juvenile Diabetes Research Foundation (JDRF) is to find a cure for type 1 and type 2 diabetes. Until they do, research continues on a number of levels to develop new and innovative products and medications that will prevent, delay, and treat diabetes and its complications. In this chapter, I will discuss treatments and products currently under investigation for clients with type 1 and type 2. With type 1 diabetes, the problem concerns the autoimmune destruction of the beta cells in the islets of Langerhans of the pancreas. A cure might involve preventing or stopping this destruction or transplanting a pancreas or islet cells to restore the production of insulin.

RESEARCH IN THE PREVENTION AND CURE OF TYPE 1 DIABETES

Prevention of Autoimmune Destruction

Alba Therapeutics is conducting trials of an oral medication called AT-1001, a zonulin inhibitor, that may prevent intestinal permeability caused by excessive amounts of the human protein zonulin. Increased permeability of the intestinal wall allows undigested foodstuff, toxins, and other bacterial and viral particles access to the immune system which can lead to the production of antibodies that can destroy the insulin-producing islet cells of the pancreas among people genetically predisposed to developing type 1 diabetes (Fasano, 2005). If this medication is given to patients in the earliest stages of type 1, it might halt the process and preserve beta cell function. Another potential drug to halt autoimmune destruction is an anti-CD3 monoclonal antibody infused over several days in clients with recent-onset type 1 diabetes. In a recent clinical trial, this short-term treatment preserved residual beta cell function for at least 2 years (Herold et al., 2005).

The researchers at the Juvenile Diabetes Research Foundation (JDRF) Center working on immunological tolerance in type 1 diabetes at Harvard Medical School have found the genetic region that usually stops errant T cells of the immune system from attacking the body's tissue, such as the beta cell. The immune system, which protects the body from *non-self* invaders such as bacteria and viruses also sometimes release *misguided* T cells, which have the potential to attack the body's own cells. There is a safeguard mechanism, a process called tolerance, that should find and destroy such errant T cells. However, in people with autoimmune diseases, such as type 1 diabetes, rheumatoid arthritis, multiple sclerosis, types of hypo- and hyperthyroidism, and others, the immune system's safeguard mechanism is defective. Thus, these errant T cells seek out the body's tissue genetically marked for destruction, such as the pancreas's beta cells, and kill them. The JDRF researchers are now looking for the precise genes that control this safeguard mechanism. Once the genes are identified, procedures to *fix* the defect can be developed to prevent or halt this process of destruction (Keymeulen, 2005). The number of people with the genetic predisposition for autoimmune diseases could benefit enormously from this discovery.

The journal *Immunity,* in July 2004, published a series of experiments conducted by scientists from various research centers around the world that worked in a different way to prevent the immune system from attacking its own cells. During their research they discovered a transcription factor, PPAR-gamma, in the dendritic cells, the immature immune cells. When rosiglitazone (Avandia), a drug already used with type 2 diabetes to increase insulin sensitivity, was added to these dendritic cells, PPAR-gamma activity was increased, which activated natural killer T (NKT) cells. The researchers working on this project believe that this drug used in this manner can increase the immune system's recognition and tolerance of self, thus preventing autoimmune destruction of cells like the insulin-producing beta cells. PPAR-gamma also regulates the expression of a gene called CD1d, which encodes a glycoprotein responsible for the presentation of self and foreign lipids to T cells (Szatmari et al., 2004, p. 95). By continuing to study the PPAR-gamma pathway in non-obese diabetic mice and its effects on the CD1d gene and natural killer T cells, the hope is that this autoimmune process can be prevented or at least halted.

Transplantation

Pancreas and kidney transplantations have been performed successfully for several years. The downside to any transplantation is the potential complication of immunologic suppression needed to prevent rejection of the transplanted organs. This is currently a lifelong suppression that results in the recipient being very susceptible to infections, illnesses, and cancers. Therefore, it is only done as a last resort in selected individuals. Moreover, there is always the possibility of rejection despite the potent, daily, and expensive immunosuppressive drug cocktails. This is not of great hope for type 1 diabetics, as the cure may be worse than the disease.

What about islet cells transplantation? In 1974 the first human islet cell transplantations were performed. This therapy has had minimal success for years because some of the immunosuppressant drugs, namely corticosteroids, actually destroy the islets. To understand the process of islet cell transplantation it may be useful to point out some insulin physiology. Insulin produced by the pancreatic beta cells is not in a form the body can use. It is sometimes called *proinsulin* and must be sent to the liver where the C-peptide amino acid chain is cleaved off, leaving the A and B chains. This insulin is now ready for distribution to the body via the blood vessels. Proof that the body is producing insulin can be found by testing the blood for C-peptide amino acid chains. Because insulin produced by islet cells must first go to the liver, it makes sense to inject islet cell transplants directly into the liver instead of the pancreas. Islet cell transplantation using the Edmonton Protocol (Edmonton, Canada) has been at least 50% successful since its inception in 2000. What makes this procedure work has to do with the drugs used to prevent rejection. By omitting any corticosteroids that destroy islet cells and raise blood pressure and cholesterol levels, islet cells are preserved and continue to function for years. The immunosuppressant drugs used with the Edmonton Protocol include sirolimus, which negates the need for steroids and decreases the dose of the second drug, tacrolimus. Tacrolimus can raise blood pressure and ultimately be toxic to kidneys. It is also toxic to islet cells (Dinsmoor, 2005). The third drug, daclizumab, is used only for a short period of time to prevent initial rejection of the islet cells. Because type 1 diabetes is an autoimmune disease, immunosuppression is needed to protect the islet cells as well as to prevent rejection (Saudek & Margolis, 2006).

Islet cell transplantation is usually done in a hospital where a large number of prepared islet cells are transfused into the portal vein of the liver under the guidance of ultrasound technology. Today, islet cells are usually recovered from a cadaver pancreas and cultivated to ensure viability. As many as 300,000 islet cells are infused in a single procedure. Because this is not a major surgical procedure, clients recover in a regular hospital room and usually go home the next day. Most clients still need to take progressively lower doses of insulin to maintain normal blood sugars. The goal of islet cell transplantation is to achieve normal blood sugar without using injectable insulin. Currently, in order to achieve that goal, clients need one to three procedures of islet cell infusions, each using the islet cells from yet another cadaver pancreas (Shapiro et al., 2000).

In most of the earlier trials, it took islet cells from as many as three cadaver pancreases injected into the liver of a type 1 diabetic to produce sufficient insulin to make them insulin independent. Because there is a scarcity of cadaver pancreases and each person may need the islet cells from three, the focus now is on reducing the number of islet cells needed. Some of the methods to do this include:

1. using living matching donors
2. refining the immunosuppressant with the goal of weaning recipients off at least some of the drugs over a few years
3. salvaging functioning islet cells from the patient's own pancreas and reimplanting them in the liver thus removing the need for immunosuppressant drugs altogether
4. producing insulin secreting cells from stem cells or liver cells (Hering et al., 2005)

In January 2005, researchers from Japan successfully reversed a woman's type 1 diabetes by transplanting islet cells from the pancreas of a matching living donor. Because healthy pancreases usually have four times the beta cells needed on a daily basis, removing some, in this case, islet cells, from half of the donor's pancreas reduces the number needed by the recipient and increases the supply so that many more type 1 diabetics can be served. Islet cells from living donors improve the outcome because they are more viable and more likely to function properly over a longer period of time compared to cadaver islet cells (Matsumoto et al., 2005).

Another means of increasing transplanted islet cell survival and longevity is to prevent the initial inflammatory reaction triggered by the tissue factors of the islet cells. One drug that is being used is the antioxidant nicotinamide. If more islet cells survived transplantation, fewer would be needed. Researchers from Europe suggest that islet cells be cultured in the antioxidant nicotinamide prior to transplantation and that patients be given oral nicotinamide prior to the procedure to block tissue-factor–mediated inflammatory response to the islet cell transplants (Johansson, 2005).

Transplanting a patient's own islet cells (autologous transplantation) has been performed by the University of Illinois Medical Center in Chicago where a pancreas had to be removed due to chronic pancreatitis. This removal would have caused surgical diabetes and the patient would have required insulin as well as pancreatic enzyme replacement for life. By isolating the patient's own islet cells from his removed pancreas and reinjecting them into the liver, the client's insulin production was resumed. This could potentially also be done in the early stages of type 1 diabetes prior to significant beta cell destruction.

Beta Cell Regeneration

This new field, beta cell regeneration, is based on getting beta cells of the pancreas to reproduce themselves to replace those cells lost through aging or disease. This would provide no limit to the number of beta cells an individual could produce, which would eliminate two of the most troublesome difficulties with islet cell transplantation, namely, shortages of islet cell donors and the need for immunosuppressive drugs. If the beta cells in mice replicate themselves, why cannot humans do it?

In November 2004, researchers at the National Institutes of Health (NIH) caused human pancreatic cells to revert to a more primitive form so they could multiply and produce islet cells that produced insulin. The drawback was that these cells produced far less insulin than the original beta cells. The fact that this replication could happen at all ensures continued research on this topic.

Would it not be wonderful if type 1 diabetics could grow their own beta cells to replace those destroyed by their errant immune system? Another interesting fact discovered early in 2005 was that the majority of type 1 diabetics, even those with long-standing diabetes, continue to form insulin-producing beta cells (Juvenile Diabetes Research Foundation, 2005). Now all we have to do is stop the autoimmune destruction and find ways to increase beta cell replication to return the insulin production back to normal.

Oral Insulin

Insulin cannot be given orally because the digestive enzymes of the stomach and intestines destroy it before it can be absorbed into the bloodstream. Or so it has been taught. Nobex Corporation is working on an oral dose of a modified human insulin for clients with type 1 and type 2 diabetes. Hexyl-insulin monoconjugate 2 (HIM2) is an orally active insulin that is in Phase II clinical development. Orally delivered insulin follows the same pathway into the body as does natural insulin secreted by the pancreas, through portal vein directly into the liver. Results from Phase I and Phase II clinical studies to date demonstrate that oral insulin (1) has showed no significant side effects; (2) acts to lower glucose; and (3) shows the ability to stabilize or lower blood glucose in proportion to the amount of drug given, thus decreasing the risk of hypoglycemia. This chemically altered insulin is part of a polymer drug molecule that makes it resistant to enzyme activity of the stomach and small intestine. This insulin is fast-acting and could replace mealtime insulin injections. Nobex is now testing a newer oral insulin called IN-105, which may hold up to digestive enzymes even better than HIM2 does.

Nobex Corporation filed for Chapter 11 bankruptcy protection on December 1, 2005, however, it is actively marketing its intellectual properties, which include IN-105. Other companies are also working on oral insulin, namely Diabetology (http://www.diabetology.co.uk/projects.htm) and Emisphere (http://www.emisphere.com/pc_oi.asp). Hopefully progress in developing an oral insulin product will continue and someday insulin can be administered orally. For more information on oral insulin, a search for "oral insulin" on the Internet should provide data on its current development.

RESEARCH IN THE PREVENTION AND CURE
OF TYPE 2 DIABETES

The causes of type 2 diabetes include insulin resistance mediated by genetics and obesity. The focus of current research seems to be on prevention, diagnosis, and reversing the components of metabolic syndrome that occur in so many clients with type 2 diabetes. The diagnosis of metabolic syndrome is made when at least three out of five of the following characteristics are present.

1. a waist circumference greater than 40 inches in men and 35 inches in women
2. triglyceride levels greater than 150 mg/dl
3. HDL cholesterol less than 40 mg/dl in men or 50 mg/dl in women
4. blood pressure of 130/85 mm Hg or higher, or taking any antihypertensive drugs
5. fasting glucose levels of 110 mg/dl or higher (Saudek & Margolis, 2006)

A recent study found that 27% of Americans (more than one in four) over the age of 20 have been diagnosed with metabolic syndrome, up from 24% in a study from the early to middle 1990s. The greatest increase was in women whose waist circumference, blood pressure, and triglycerides accounted for the increased diagnosis (Ford, Giles, & Mokdad, 2004). With all of the factors involved in metabolic syndrome, the greatest threat these factors pose for type 2 diabetics is for cardiovascular compromise. Much of the research is focused on new drugs and combinations of drugs to combat the various characteristics of this insidious syndrome.

HOW A NEW DRUG OR PRODUCT GETS APPROVED

With almost 21 million people with diabetes, it is big business. Pharmaceutical and manufacturing companies take this target consumer population very seriously. Scores of new antidiabetic drugs, including new insulins, and unique deliveries of such medication as well as treatments for diabetic complications are under investigation as you read this book. Many never come to market, such as the nasal insulin of 10 years ago. Some take decades, such as the now promising inhaled insulin. Some, after considerable experimentation, get FDA approved only to be recalled due to adverse reaction, such as the first glitazone on the market, Rezulin. The process from development to availability involves many phases, some of which involve healthy individuals as well as those who have the disease.

Prior to investigational trials using human subjects, scientists research new treatments in test tubes and experiment on animals, usually mice or rats, to test hypotheses about the potential use of this or that chemical combination. If they discover a promising chemical compound to treat any number of potential causes of a disease or its complications, they refine the process and then may move on to larger animals. After more refinement as to dosage, timing, method of delivery, safety, and side effect profiles, they may start clinical trials using human subjects. Phase I uses small numbers of healthy, paid adult volunteers of both genders and most races to test the effects of an experimental drug or treatment to further refine safety, dose range, and side effects, and to evaluate whether there are unintended consequences in humans such as liver, kidney, or other potential problems. The subjects are evaluated often and are taken off the protocols if any negative reactions occur.

If all goes well in Phase I, the drug or treatment goes into Phase II. This usually occurs in a few research medical centers and involves a small number of clients with the disease, in this case, type 1 or type 2 diabetes. These paid volunteers must meet certain criteria. They usually receive free exams, care, and experimental medication or treatment to get a better drug or treatment profile and to see if the experimental treatment works as intended in human subjects for which it was developed. A further refinement of safety issues and dosage also occurs. This may take weeks or months, but in the end, the drug or treatment is ready for Phase III or is scrapped and returned to the drawing board. Those drugs or treatments that get to Phase III are tested in double- or triple-blind clinical trials at medical centers across the country and worldwide involving large numbers of volunteers for which the experimental drug or treatment was intended. The subjects are divided into a control group, which may be given a placebo or current therapy, and an experimental group receiving the item to be tested. This phase compares the experimental treatment with currently available treatments and/or placebo. Neither the volunteers nor those conducting the experiment know who is receiving either the investigational therapy or a placebo to prevent the placebo effect. (The placebo effect is when the client expects something to happen and it does, even though the client was not on the *real* medication.)

TABLE 6.1   Four Phases of Investigational Drug Studies

PHASE I

Small numbers of healthy volunteers (as opposed to volunteers afflicted with the disease or ailment that the drug is meant to treat). Purpose is to determine the optimal dosage and pharmacokinetics of the drug (absorption, distribution, metabolism, excretion). Tests are performed.

PHASE II

Small numbers of volunteers that have the disease or ailment that the drug is designed to diagnose or treat. Participants are monitored for drug effectiveness and side effect. If *none* may proceed to III.

PHASE III

Involves a large numbers of patients at medical research centers. Large numbers provide information about frequent or rare adverse effects that have been identified in small group study. Placebos are used to prevent bias. Study is blinded investigational so investigator does not know which group has the actual drug being tested (double-blind or placebo-controlled study objectives are clinical effectiveness, safety, and dosage range).

NEW DRUG APPLICATION

At this point the FDA reviews all result the company may submit in the new drug application. If approved the company is free to market the drug exclusively.

PHASE IV

Postmarketing studies voluntarily conducted to gain further proof of therapeutic effects of new drug. (When drugs are used in the general population sometimes severe adverse effects show up.)

Everything is numbered, and records are evaluated by a third party not involved in the actual experiment. Volunteers receive frequent free care, treatment, and instructions; records are kept; and the length of the trial is variable from weeks to months to years. Volunteers may be lost to follow-up or taken off the protocol due to unforeseen occurrences that may or may not have anything to do with the experimental treatment. However, the trial subject numbers are so large that it really does not alter the data. Only after all of the data from animal studies through Phase III are completed is a new drug application (NDA) submitted to the U.S. Food and Drug Administration (FDA). The FDA evaluates the drug and either approves, approves provisionally, or rejects it. At any time along this path an idea may be stopped, reformulated, or continued. Once an experimental drug or treatment has been

FDA approved, it enters Phase IV, where it can be prescribed to patients fitting the criteria for which it was designed. At this point, prescribers are still
submitting data on side effects and other information from the clients using
this newly approved drug. This phase may go on for years and may lead to
a drug being taken off the market if there are reports of significant adverse
reactions, such as with Rezulin, which caused liver damage.

Volunteering to be a clinical trial participant can significantly impact
the course of treatment for diabetes or any other disease or condition. Dis-
ease-free individuals are usually recruited for Phase I trials and those with
the disease for Phase II and III. Most clients are involved in Phase III.
See Table 6.1 for a summary of the phases of investigational drug studies.
There is a detailed informed consent involved that does not bind the vol-
unteer to remain in the study. To learn more about new and ongoing clinical trials and participant criteria, visit the National Institute of Diabetes
and Digestive and Kidney Diseases' (NIDDK) home page at http://www.
niddk.nih.gov/patient/patientdiabetes.htm and click on "Diabetes Clinical
Research." You can also check out http://www.clinicaltrials.gov for clinical trials by location and condition being studied.

REFERENCES

Clark, W. L. (2005, Spring). As islet transplant success grows, organ trans-
plants continue to save lives. *JDRF Countdown,* pp. 31–39.
Dinsmoor, R. S. (2005, Spring). Rebooting the immune system. *JDRF
Countdown,* pp. 8–17.
Fasano, A. (2005, February 22). Potential method for preventing type 1
diabetes. *Proceedings of the National Academy of Sciences, USA.*
Ford, E. S., Giles, W. H., & Mokdad, A. H. (2004). Increasing prevalence
of the metabolic syndrome among U.S. adults. *Diabetes Care, 27,*
2444–2449.
Hering, B. J., Kandaswamy, R., Ansite, J. D., Eckman, P. M., Nakano, M.,
Sawada, T., et al. (2005, February 16). Single-donor, marginal-dose islet
transplantation in pations with type 1 diabetes. *Journal of the American
Medical Association, 293,* 830–835.
Herold, K. C., Gitelman, S. E., Masharani, U., Hagopian, W.,
Bisikirska, B., Donaldson, D., et al. (2005). A single course of anti-CD3
monoclonal antibody hOKT3γ1(Ala-Ala) results in improvement in

C-peptide responses and clinical parameters for at least 2 years after onset of type 1 diabetes. *Diabetes, 54,* 1763–1769.

Juvenile Diabetes Research Foundation. (2005, Spring). Researchers make strides in understanding beta cell regeneration. *Discoveries,* p. 5.

Johansson, H. (2005). Blocking tissue factor-mediated inflammatory response may improve islet cell engraftment. *Diabetes, 54,* 1755–1762.

Keymeulen, B. (2005). CD3 antibodies may be helpful in recent-onset type 1 diabetes. *New England Journal of Medicine, 352,* 2598–2608, 2642–2644.

Mathis, D., & Benoist, C. (2005, March). Genetic defect in immunologic tolerance. *Immunity, 22,* 385–396.

Matsumoto, S., Okitsu T., Iwanaga Y., Noguchi H., Nagata H., Yonekawa Y., et al. (2005, May 7). Insulin independence after living-donor distal pancreatectomy and islet cell allotransplantation. *Lancet, 365,* 1642–1644.

Saudek, C. D., & Margolis, S. (2006). *Johns Hopkins white papers: Diabetes.* Redding, CT: Medletter Associates.

Shapiro, A. M. J., Lakey, J. R. T., Ryan, E. A., Korbutt, G. S., Toth, E., Warnock, G. L., et al. (2000, July 27). Islet transplantation in seven patients with type 1 diabetes mellitus using a glucocorticoid-free immunosuppressive regimen. *New England Journal of Medicine, 343,* 230–238.

Szatmari, I., Gogolak, P., Im, J. S., Dezso, B., Rajnavolgyi, E., & Nagy, L. (2004, July). Activation of PPARγ specifies a dendritic cell subtype capable of enhanced induction of iNKT cell expansion. *Immunity, 21,* 95–106.

Part II

Diabetes Self-Management

What I wanted most as a newly diagnosed diabetic was a set of rules to help me live with this chronic illness. As I left the doctor's office that day of diagnosis, I wondered what in the world I could fix for dinner that evening. Because I was never an inpatient, I did not have the luxury of having a consultation with a registered dietitian. So I bought a diabetic cookbook. By dinnertime I had decided that what we usually ate was going to have to do. At my next office visit, I asked to see a dietitian and was told my insurance would not cover this as an outpatient. I told my doctor that he had two choices. He could teach me what I needed to know about my diet or he could request a dietary consult. So for the grand total of $16 an hour I sat with first one, then a second registered dietitian, learned the standard instruction, and then picked their brains for rationale and "what ifs" and got my questions answered. It occurred to me then that if I had not insisted on getting someone to teach me what I needed to know, I might still be floundering and overwhelmed. The second thing that occurred to me after this experience was that the rest of my education was up to me. What a scary thought, but at least I had a head start.

After about a year and a half into my career as a diabetic, a wonderful thing happened. I was asked, along with many others with type 1 and type 2 diabetes, to participate in a research project to see if diabetics could be trained to be better guessers of blood sugars, both high and low. At that point glucose monitors were just becoming popular and affordable (but not small and not covered by insurance yet). I jumped at the opportunity. Toward the end of the 6 weeks, the participants and I were communicating with each other more than the researchers were. I asked if the other participants wanted to continue to meet as a support group. The response was overwhelming. Because *I* needed a support group and there was none in my area, I started one. I led this group for 7 years, well after it had met my personal needs. I learned how desperate people and their families were for any advice, education, and opportunities to share their stories. This all came about by dumb luck, but if it weren't for dumb luck, some of us would have no luck at all.

I hope that the chapters in this section of the book inspire nurses to use opportunities to teach peers and clients alike what they desperately need and want to know about how to live with this chronic illness that affects every minute of their lives. How you respond to their questions, their silence, their sarcasm, even their noncompliance will let them know if you are the one that they can finally talk to. Maybe their dumb luck is having you as their nurse.

7

The Nurse as Teacher

The roots of true achievement lie in the will to become the best that you can become.

Harold Taylor

Nurses wear many hats, perform many functions, and fulfill many roles. These facts contribute to our immense value and also to our great challenge. In my view, the most important impact nurses can make on any client and his or her family is to teach them how to promote health and prevent illness. I believe in the old saying, "If you give a man a fish, you feed him for a day. If you teach him how to fish, you feed him for a lifetime."

The American Diabetes Association, in its 2006 *"Standards of Medical Care in Diabetes,"* states, "Diabetes is a chronic illness that requires continuing medical care and patient self-management education to prevent acute complications and reduce the risk of long-term complications. Diabetes care is complex and requires that many issues, beyond glycemic control, be addressed" (ADA, 2006, p. S5).

Nursing students are all taught the importance of client teaching. They may have written care plans or care paths concerning client teaching needs and interventions. As busy clinicians, however, the more objective clinical skills seem to matter most. Unless we have a physician's order for "diabetic teaching," it is easy to overlook this very important aspect of client care. Nurses may make assumptions about what clients know based on how many years they have lived with the disease. They may reinforce behaviors when clients choose "correct" foods on the menu or give insulin appropriately. However, most nurses administer insulin and other medications that clients and/or their families give at home without even asking them about this part of their overall self-care. Patients who complain, ask too many questions, or who are demanding may be labeled as "difficult" or worse. When blood sugars are too high, nurses may assume they are "cheating" or noncompliant.

I once asked a thirty-something type 1 diabetic, who I assigned to one of my clinical students, why she thought her fasting blood sugars were so high. She started crying and stated that she was not "cheating" or guilty of the other accusations nurses and doctors had made since her admission. After explaining that she was the recipient of a transplanted kidney, that her sight was deteriorating, and that her ultimate goal was to live long enough to experience her only child's graduation from high school, she looked at me and said, "Why would I jeopardize that by eating candy?" So I started from scratch and did an assessment of her insulin regimen at home. The answer to the puzzle of high fasting blood sugars became obvious when the mixed dose of regular and NPH insulins she took at home before dinner was not carried out in the hospital. She was only getting regular insulin prior to dinner. Not only was she a type 1 diabetic with virtually no basal insulin being produced by her own pancreas, but she was also taking antirejection medications, including prednisone and cyclosporine, both of which elevate blood sugar. At my urging, her nurse called the physician, who promptly added NPH to her evening dose. This interaction took me a maximum of 10 minutes. Afterwards, I was upset with myself that I had not done this a few days earlier when I first learned of the problem. I allowed myself to believe the "cheating" scenario without first investigating or questioning the reporting nurses about the facts that had led them to this conclusion. Because nurses drew up the client's insulin in the medication room and administered it to her, the client never realized the error, and the nurses, including me, never questioned the inappropriate lack of a second dose of NPH with the evening meal for this patient. This was an important lesson for me about giving care without appropriate and individualized assessment data.

WHAT DO CLIENTS WITH DIABETES NEED TO KNOW?

Before nurses can impact diabetes self-management, we need to have a clear understanding of exactly what someone with diabetes needs to know in order to take care of himself or herself. Redman (2004, p. 66) lists the following self-management tasks required to successfully control diabetes:

1. self-monitoring blood glucose levels
2. daily medications (insulin and/or oral agents)

3. nutrition—eating regularly and controlling weight
4. regular physical exercise
5. recognizing early symptoms of hypo- or hyperglycemia and responding appropriately
6. adapting medication dose and timing to account for blood sugar levels, food intake, and activity level
7. checking feet regularly for lesions
8. getting frequent blood pressure and cholesterol checks
9. getting periodic eye and renal function tests

Of these tasks, the first five are crucial and should be taught with the initial diagnosis and reviewed with each client encounter. The other behaviors can be added to what is discussed with the client if time permits or at a later date if the client is seen regularly. In Table 7.1, the American Diabetes Association differentiates between survival skills and daily management issues. Many clients cope with the threat to their health that a new diagnosis brings with a desire to do their own research. In their research, clients should be directed to these most important organizations: the American Diabetes Association (ADA), http://www.diabetes.org, and the Juvenile Diabetes Research Foundation (JDRF), http://www.jdrf.org.

TABLE 7.1　Major Components of Diabetes Self-Management Education

Survival skills	Daily management issues
• Hypo-/hyperglycemia	• Disease process
• Sick day management	• Nutritional management
• Medication	• Physical activity
• Monitoring	• Medications
• Foot care	• Monitoring
	• Acute complications
	• Risk reduction
	• Goal setting/problem solving
	• Psychosocial adjustment
	• Preconception care/pregnancy/gestational diabetes management

Note. From "Diabetes Management in Correctional Institutions," *Diabetes Care, 29,* p. S63. Copyright © 2006 by the American Diabetes Association. Reprinted with permission from the American Diabetes Association.

ASSESSMENT GUIDELINES

We all know that assessment is the first step of the nursing process. Most acute care institutions have a multipage patient questionnaire that is completed by the admitting nurse. Some of the data are collected in an objective format with yes/no answers from the client and/or family. In addition, it includes a list of medications with dosages and times, but it should also include space for questions about who administers the drugs, the timing with regard to other meds and food, the client's knowledge of the drug's purpose, and his or her thoughts concerning its effectiveness. These follow-up questions ought to be asked and charted whether or not there is a line for such responses on the questionnaire. However, even the best assessment data are only good if they are read and used by every nurse who delivers care to this individual. If generic care plans are not modified to individualize the nursing care, then such assessment tools serve only to meet Joint Commission on Accreditation of Healthcare Organizations (JCAHO) requirements and those of other agencies but do not help meet the client's or family's needs. Perhaps if this assessment form were placed in front of the patient's chart, more nurses would read it and use the information more appropriately in their care for the client.

GOALS OF CLIENT EDUCATION

Identifying goals or expected outcomes is paramount in planning care for clients. "The overriding goal of patient education should be to support the patient's autonomous decision making, not (as it has been conceptualized) to get the patients to follow doctor's orders.... True patient autonomy requires creating new options to meet patient needs, not just as is now frequently the case, having the right to refuse a treatment option" (Redman, 2004, p. 7). Although I agree with Redman's client-centered approach, I wish the author had used the word "client" instead of "patient." I have used the two terms interchangeably throughout this book; however, when discussing autonomy and decision making, it seems imperative to use the word client. In order to increase client autonomy in our pattern of health care delivery, we all need to view individuals and families who seek health care as people with options. They should be able to freely choose which health care providers, health care facilities, and health care management systems best suit their needs and values. This should give them the power to change providers or refuse to follow any part or all of the medical management provided. Most people would agree with this, yet when I attempted to practice autonomous decision making a few years ago, prior to elective surgery, I met with considerable obstacles and bewilderment by health care providers. I insisted on interviewing the anesthesiologist who was scheduled to provide anesthesia during surgery to discuss my request for an epidural as opposed to general anesthesia. In addition, I also discussed my pain management requests with him. I then interviewed the unit manager where I would be transferred after surgery in order to discuss how her staff might handle occurrences having to do with high or low blood sugars. I requested my own vials of insulin to be kept at the bedside because I wanted to draw up and administer my own insulin unless I was unable to do so. I also stated that I would use my own glucose meter and have my own supply of 6-ounce cans of orange juice and glucose tablets at the bedside. My compromise with this unit manager was to report to her staff any insulin or orange juice administered and to use their meter with my own as ordered and at any other appropriate times. My diabetologist provided orders for the above to ensure that my need to be in control of my diabetes was met. My surgery and the resulting care I received were as positive an experience as possible because my anxiety level and my blood sugars were under my control. Clients with less experience than I have with health care might not be able to anticipate potential problems as I could. They also may not be as assertive. However, asking pertinent questions about how the client and/or family envision the hospital stay or agency care might help to get concerns out in the open and make them feel like they are part of the team. Questions like the following could be asked:

1. "How would you like your medications given and by whom?"

This might involve a discussion by the nurse about the purpose and timing of each medication and allowing the client or a family member to administer the medication under supervision to assess technique. Even if the client requests that the nurse give injections, the client ought to be observed doing this a few times before discharge.

2. "How do you know you are having a low blood sugar and what do you usually do about it? How would you like us to handle this?"

This might involve treating a low first and doing a blood sugar after or allowing the client to treat a low blood sugar and notify us after the fact. This would decrease the anxiety the client might have concerning delayed treatment. It could also involve a discussion of signs and symptoms and possible treatments unknown to the client. The rule of 15 (15 grams of carbohydrates, wait 15 minutes) should be taught to prevent overtreating a low blood sugar.

    3. "How often do you usually test your blood sugar? Who do you want to do them? What are the ranges of blood sugar that you aim for fasting, premeal, and at bedtime? What do you do if the blood sugar is too high at this time?"

This might involve a discussion of when blood sugars have been ordered. They may be more or less often than the client expects. If a sliding scale insulin is ordered, the client should be informed. The client may be upset that he or she might get insulin or may be dismayed that the sliding scale only starts at a blood sugar of 250 mg/dl.

    I spoke to a group of insulin pump users to which I belong and told them that I was writing this book. Before I could ask them what they wanted me to include, they all started telling me of their most recent experiences in hospitals and/or rehabilitation agencies. Most were angry that they had to either turn off their pumps and go back to shots or that their personal range for normal was disregarded. Sliding scale insulin started too high, ordered insulin doses did not account for carbohydrates in a meal or the timing of meals. In other words, they were treated as patients and felt they had no autonomy in controlling their diabetes. One person stated that his recovery from cataract surgery was delayed, not because he had diabetes, but because his diabetes was poorly managed in the hospital and that he was not consulted in developing his plan of care. He was angry at the doctors and their inadequate orders and the nurses who did not listen to his needs and good sense. "They should have called the doctor when the insulin ordered did not control my blood sugars." In other words, the nurses should have been client advocates. It is a given that most clients on insulin pumps are a special group. They test often, make multiply daily management decisions based on blood sugars, value tight control, and are very knowledgeable about how diabetes affects them. This group wanted me to encourage nurses to ask, in addition to the above three questions, the following:

    4. "Tell me how you control your blood sugar with your insulin pump? How can I assist you in doing this?"

This might involve advocating for them with the physician, who may want to discontinue pump use. It might also involve the nurse learning more about insulin pumps in general and this client and his or her pump in particular. Letting the client explain what he or she is doing and why it will serve both the nurse and client well (Chase, 2005, p. 55).

The article "Don't Take My Pump" by H. Peter Chase, MD, in the September 2005 *Diabetes Forecast* is a "must read" for any nurse who is assigned to a client on an insulin pump. In fact, this issue of *Diabetes Forecast* includes a group of articles discussing, "What You Need to Know Before Your Hospital Stay." These articles can be found at http://www.diabetes.org under *Diabetes Forecast*. Additionally, I have included a questionnaire that I used to help me write this book (see Figure 7.1). Using some of the ideas in this questionnaire could help nurses better understand the client and his or her needs.

NURSING INTERVENTIONS USING LEARNING PRINCIPLES

No matter what reason brings a client with diabetes to your outpatient or inpatient facility, you must assess and evaluate the client's understanding of diabetes self-management. In fact, if diabetes has contributed to the client's admission, this may be an opportune time to increase his or her knowledge of how to recover and prevent reoccurrence. This is what is called a *teachable moment.* You have the client's attention and can teach new information or review material he or she may have ignored in the past. The learning principles taken from my first book, *Teaching Nursing in an Associate Degree Program,* are outlined in Table 7.2. "People learn best those things that hold particular interest for them" and "learning occurs most quickly if a person can see how new information will benefit him" are particularly relevant here. The client has had a wake-up call and is eager to avoid a repeat of this incident. See Table 7.2 for other learning principles that should guide any teaching.

Anyone with diabetes who needs the care of a nurse should expect to learn more about his or her body, health, nutrition, and diabetes. That means that nurses need to stay current by attending workshops, reviewing professional journals, and reading books like this one and/or updating their knowledge periodically on the Internet. This is all part of being a professional. Some of the steps to good client-centered teaching include the following:

FIGURE 7.1 DIABETES QUESTIONNAIRE

I am writing a book about what nurses need to know about teaching patients how to manage their diabetes. I want to include as many areas of concern as possible and need your help. By completing this questionnaire, you will provide valuable input so that I can address your areas of concern adequately. I am a nursing instructor and have had diabetes for 20 years so I know some of your concerns and have included them in my diabetes discussions with student nurses. However, because the diabetes experience is so individualized and varied, I need to include a greater variety of experiences. How better to get this information than to ask you. Thank you for your assistance.

PROFILE

Age ____   Sex ____   Age at   Current   Height
                        diagnosis   weight ____   _____
                        ____

Please circle whichever applies.

Type of Diabetes:	Type 1	Type 2	Gestational	Don't know

Controlled by:	Oral Medication	Insulin	Diet and exercise	Weight loss

If on oral medication, please circle *which drug* and *list dosage* and *when taken* on line below drug:

DiaBeta	Gynase PresTab	Micronase	Amaryl	Glucotrol	Glucotrol XL
_____	_____	_____	_____	_____	_____

Glucophage	Prandin	Precose	Glyset	Actos	Avandia
_____	_____	_____	_____	_____	_____

If on insulin, please circle *kind of insulin* and *list amount* and *when taken* on line below type:

Regular	NPH	Humalog	Novolog	Lantus	Other
_____	_____	_____	_____	_____	_____

If you are following a particular diet, Please circle or write in which one.

_____   calories   Low carbo- Low fat   Low Protein Other
                        hydrate

How often do you eat a meal per day? Please circle whichever applies.

3 meals	2 meals	1 meal	Varies	Snacking only

How many snacks do you have per day? _____

How often do you exercise?_____

If you exercise, circle which of the following types of exercise you practice and state how often.

Walking   Jogging   Bicycling   Swimming   Dancing   Other

_____   _____   _____   _____   _____   _____

Do you have any diabetic complications? If so, please circle which ones and state when diagnosed.

Problems with:

Eyes   Kidneys   Heart   Legs   Nerves   Other

_____   _____   _____   _____   _____   _____

When diagnosed:

_____   _____   _____   _____   _____   _____

Please circle if you have
ever experienced   Hypoglycemia   Hyperglycemia

How often?

NURSING CARE

Have you ever been hospitalized? _____ If yes, list dates and reason.____

_____

_____

Did nurses help you understand diabetes better? _____

_____

_____

_____

Were you treated with respect? _____

_____

_____

_____

What would you have liked to know more about? _____

_____

_____

_____

If you are hospitalized in the future for a diabetic or non-diabetic related reason, what could nurses do that would make your hospitalization better?

_____

_____

_____

Developed by Rita Mertig, MS, RNC, CNS. May be duplicated for instructional purposes.

1. Before attempting to teach anyone, the nurse must assess prior knowledge and readiness to learn. Even if the client's readiness is in doubt, do something to get that person's attention. Preparing insulin in the room with the client watching while providing commentary on the necessary steps used and the rationale for each will, at least, peak his interest. Most nurses do not do that. Letting a client know that prior to discharge he or she will be expected to draw up and deliver his or her own insulin will certainly give the client a reason to pay attention to what you are doing. Building on preexisting knowledge will demonstrate your respect for the client and increase his or her self-esteem.

Giving what I call the "canned speech" ignores the client's individuality, causes resentment, and worse, may lead to the client tuning out instructions instead of listening for "pearls" that he or she did not know. By getting clients to explain their understanding of what they have learned so far, you are evaluating their interpretation for correctness and completeness. It gives you an opportunity to reward the client for his or her knowledge base, make adjustments and updates, and fill in where gaps in knowledge exist. This should be done whether the client has a lot of knowledge, none at all, or falls anywhere in between. The canned speech fits no one, is usually too limited, and is often done at discharge, which is the worse possible time to teach. Another learning principle states: "learning plateaus and time is

TABLE 7.2   Learning Principles for the Adult Learner

Learning occurs only when a person is ready to learn.

Learning occurs most quickly if a person can see how new information will benefit him.

Adults learn best when new information builds upon preexisting knowledge.

Adults learn best when rationales are explained at their cognitive level.

People learn best those things that hold particular interest for them.

People learn best by active participation.

Learning is more likely to take place in a non-stressful and accepting environment.

Learning occurs best if rewards, not penalties, are offered.

Learning ability plateaus and time is needed to process information already learned before there is interest and motivation to learn more.

Note. From *Teaching Nursing in an Associate Degree Program,* by R. G. Mertig, Springer Publishing Company, 2003, p. 71. Reprinted with permission from Springer Publishing

needed to process information already learned before there is interest and motivation to learn more," therefore, teaching should be done from admission to discharge.

Begin with a review of what the client/family already knows, move from simple to complex, and encourage questions or concerns and the need for repetition. If they have some knowledge, you may also want to start with what they really want to know, where they might be confused, or what their fears for the future are. As you gain their trust, develop a positive therapeutic relationship, and, most importantly, make them feel included in developing outcomes and planning what should be taught, it is more likely that they will learn and remember what was taught. See Figure 7.2 for a questionnaire that I have used to assess a client's attitude toward diabetes, his or her knowledge base, and what he or she thinks is most important.

2. Nurses must explain everything they do or assist clients in doing, such as giving insulin or testing blood sugars, and must give rationale for these actions at the client's cognitive level using methods that he or she has identified as ways in which he or she learns best. The client may prefer to watch videos on technical skills or read about procedures with pictures depicting each step. Handouts

FIGURE 7.2 DIABETES MELLITUS CLIENT QUESTIONNAIRE

Please complete the following sentences with as many answers that apply describing your feelings and knowledge base about diabetes.

1. I have had diabetes for _____ years/months.

2. In my opinion, diabetes is a (circle as many as apply)

challenge	opportunity	learning experience	curse	death sentence
disaster	punishment	family problem	wake-up call	
no big deal	doable	other _____		

3. I feel that my diabetes control is

terrible   improving   good   excellent

Please rate your knowledge about the following from 1–4.

1 = none   2 = minimal   3 = average   4 = very knowledgeable

4. My knowledge about diabetes is	1	2	3	4
5. My knowledge about a diabetes diet is	1	2	3	4
6. My knowledge about exercise and diabetes is	1	2	3	4
7. My knowledge about my diabetes medications is (insulin and/or pills)	1	2	3	4
8. My knowledge about high and low blood sugars is	1	2	3	4
9. My knowledge about foot care is	1	2	3	4
10. My knowledge about long-term complications is	1	2	3	4
11. My knowledge about blood sugars is	1	2	3	4
12. My family's knowledge of diabetes is	1	2	3	4

13. With regard to controlling my blood sugars, I would describe myself as

motivated	discouraged	confused	aggressive	apathetic
compulsive	fatalistic	don't care	angry	optimistic

14. Most of my information about diabetes comes from

_____

_____

15. I would like to know more about

_____

_____

16. What would help me the most to improve my diabetes control would be

_____

_____

17. The biggest problem I have in controlling my diabetes is

_____

_____

18. I would like my health care provider (MD, nurse practitioner, diabetes educator) to

_____

_____

19. I learn best with (circle as many as apply)

| discussion | written material | computer material | videos |
| demonstra-tion | hands-on | support group | audio tapes |

20. I would describe my self-management of diabetes as (circle only one)

nonexistent   following the rules   hard work   part of living

21. What worries me the most about having diabetes is

_____

_____

22. My idea of a good blood sugar is

_____ before   _____ before dinner   _____ at bedtime
breakfast

23. Diabetes has affected my life by

_____

_____

reinforce what has been taught, increase a client's sense of self-confidence, and reduce anxiety, as the client can take written material home as reference material. Many clients prefer to watch a live demonstration several times and then redemonstrate with guidance until they feel confident that they can perform the task on their own. This cannot be done adequately on the day of discharge.

3. Because "people learn best by active participation," involving the client in redemonstrating skills or repeating signs and symptoms of hypo- and hyperglycemia as well as actions that should be taken when these occur helps to solidify what has been taught. Using a client's past experiences can provide an occasion to praise the client for good problem solving when things went well or help the client to rethink his or her decisions to better resolve a similar situation in the future.

Problem solving is often one of the most difficult skills to teach, and yet it is the key to appropriate and effective self-management. Redman (2004) recounts a study of a low-income, inner-city population, comparing those with good disease control to those with poor control. They all had similar problems, complaints, and concerns about their disease state; however, "Those in good control showed good problem-solving skills, reflected a positive orientation toward diabetes SM [self-management], and a rational problem-solving process, and actively used past experience to solve current problems" (Redman, 2004, pp. 67–69).

4. Timing is everything. "Learning is more likely to take place in a non-stressful and accepting environment," so make sure the client is not in pain or worried about a test or procedure unless what you teach will decrease the client's anxiety. Simply asking if this is a good time to discuss a topic demonstrates respect and sets the stage for a positive interaction. Make sure it is truly a discussion with input from the client and/or family and not just another lecture. If it is never a good time for a certain client, then the approach might be, "Mr. Smith, we need to discuss how your medication works. Would you like to do this before or after breakfast (or shower, or whatever)?" This way you give the client options you can live with. As stated above, the day of discharge is the worst possible time because the client is too distracted. However, the client's knowledge acquired since admission should be reviewed at that time.

5. Ask the client what he or she would like to learn first or most. "Learning occurs most quickly if a person can see how new information will benefit him," so providing a short list and letting the client set the agenda, including questions and concerns, allows you to tailor

your information to the client's specific learning needs at this time in his or her life. Giving a client some real-life scenarios to ponder will help him or her to use what he or she already knows or has just learned in new and different ways. Ask questions like, "What would you do if you realized that you were having a bad low blood sugar?" The client may have a ready answer, or you may need to help the client plan for such an event by suggesting that he or she always have a fast-acting, simple sugar with him or her. A follow-up question might be, "What if this happened when you were driving?"

6. Another area of concern may be the financial impact of the cost of medication and supplies. If this is not expressed by the client, ask, "What would you do if you realized you were going to run out of your diabetes medication before you received you next paycheck?" It would be important for you to help the client troubleshoot this potential problem. Consequences of not taking the appropriate dose of medication due to cost need to be emphasized, and a new approach needs to be thought out, from borrowing money to getting a partial refill from the pharmacist until the client can pay for the rest. The client may also qualify for free or reduced-cost drugs from the many companies that offer such assistance. Refer the client to the Partnership for Prescription Assistance at http://pparx.org. See chapter 4 for a list of Web sites related to patient assistance.

7. "Learning occurs best if rewards, not penalties, are offered." Praise goes a long way in reinforcing positive behavior at any age. Evaluating a client's responses to questions and his contribution to the discussion in a positive manner will increase his or her self-esteem and sense of accomplishment. Thank the client and his family for their attention. Make an appointment with them to continue the discussion and work on other learning needs.

EVALUATING TEACHING

Teaching is never completed until learning has been evaluated. Until this is done, we have no idea whether our teaching efforts were successful. Learning is best demonstrated by a change in behavior, ability, or attitude. If a client learns what was taught, he or she has become someone different from who he or she was before. By asking questions, we can evaluate how a client feels about himself or herself and his or her ability to cope with chronic illness.

When I became a participant in the research group described at the beginning of part 2, I was asked how I felt about my diabetes. Some of the options included: crisis, catastrophe, curse, death sentence, demoralizing, disaster; as well as challenge, opportunity, new beginning, learning experience, wake-up call, no big deal, doable. Although I chose "disaster" to describe how I felt about my life with diabetes that first day, I changed it to "challenge" at the end of the 6 weeks. I had learned so much about how to tell if my blood sugar was high or low that I felt I could learn to control this disease and still live the life I wanted to live. My attitude and my outlook had been changed thanks to the knowledge I had acquired.

With short stays in an acute care facility, the behavior change that you would be able to evaluate might not be so dramatic, but getting the client to choose between some of the options I listed above would give you an idea where of he or she is at this point as opposed to where he or she was on admission. At discharge, asking if the client felt he or she had a better handle on diabetes self-management might indicate growth. Other means of evaluating learning have already been discussed, such as return demonstrations of glucose monitoring or insulin injections and asking for symptoms of hypo- or hyperglycemia. Questions about when the client would call the doctor or dial 911 might evaluate his or her knowledge of what is serious as opposed to what he or she could handle. Asking questions about food choices and how the client might fit in food items important to him or her would give you both some idea of how important the client feels nutrition is to his or her overall well-being. It can be as simple as asking, "What do you intend to change about your diabetes self-care at home?" "What have you learned while you were here that might prevent your returning?" or "In what way has the information you have received changed you?" You may find that your goals and the client's goals were incompatible, not met, or only partially met. At this point it is time to reassess. Ask about what could have been done or said differently; what was missing? What needed more time or more practice? Then refer the client to diabetes Web sites, a diabetes educator, and/or give him or her written material, whatever is appropriate for this client. Encourage clients and their families to join the American Diabetes Association. Part of the fee pays for the very informative *Diabetes Forecast,* which helps increase self-management skills, keeps clients updated on new drugs, new tests, and new dietary guidelines, and includes recipes and all sorts of appropriate information for anyone along the road to living life to the fullest despite having diabetes. Obviously, evaluation of learning is an ongoing process and is not best achieved as the client heads out the door. It is also a great way to evaluate your own skills at teaching diabetes self-management. If something works well, continue to use it with other clients and add variations to your teaching methodology so that you can adapt it to different clients. On the other hand, if something is not working after several tries with different individuals, then change it or look for a new approach. No one is perfect, and some clients really do not want to learn to take care of this disease or at least not at this time. Either way, it should always be considered a growth opportunity and should be valued.

Most of what I have read in preparation to write this chapter was written for advance practice nurses. Yet how many clients have an opportunity to sit down with a nurse practitioner or diabetes educator? Most clients with diabetes and their families encounter nurses at the doctor's office or clinic and often in acute care and long-term facilities. How much better served would they be if each nurse were as knowledgeable as possible about diabetes care and willing to use the steps of the nursing process to individualize teaching? The immediate and long-term learning needs of clients who have to live with and make decisions every day concerning this chronic illness would more likely be met. We need to provide the tools of self-management for our clients so they can stay healthy. Working ourselves out of a job *is* our job.

REFERENCES

American Diabetes Association. (2006). Standards of medical care in diabetes—2006. *Diabetes Care, 29,* S4–S42.

Chase, P. (2005, September). Don't take my pump. *Diabetes Forecast, 58*(9), 55–58.

Mertig, R. G. (2003). *Teaching nursing in an associate degree program.* New York: Springer.

Redman, B. K. (2004). *Advances in patient education.* New York: Springer.

8

Children With Diabetes and Their Parents

Kearsten Mauney

Parents learn a lot from their children about coping with life.

Muriel Spark

WHAT IS IT LIKE TO HAVE A CHILD WITH DIABETES?

It was the middle of January when Kearsten started to wonder what was wrong with her 2-year-old son, Brennan. He was frequently soaking his diaper. In addition to that, he would stand at the refrigerator with his hand on the door screaming, "I'm thirsty, Mommy! I'm thirsty." It took about a week of this continuing behavior for Kearsten to suspect the worst—that Brennan had diabetes. Kearsten's ex-husband was a diabetic, and she knew that the signs of frequent urination and excessive thirst were classic symptoms. At first, she tried to ignore the signs, thinking it was just a phase her son was going through. However, over the course of the second week, Brennan seemed to be getting worse. She noticed her son's jeans were getting very loose, and his complexion was poor. Finally, she couldn't ignore the signs anymore.

Kearsten took Brennan to the doctor on a Thursday afternoon. She told the doctor of his symptoms and that Brennan had had a stomach virus right after Christmas. The doctor said he would run some tests, but he doubted Brennan had diabetes. After all, he was only 2, and that was awfully early for children to be diagnosed with diabetes. Kearsten went home, hoping she was wrong and that it was something minor. But on Saturday morning, she received a phone call from the doctor. Her worst fears had come true; Brennan's blood sugar was in the 200s, and he had diabetes. Kearsten was told he needed to go to the hospital right away. Her doctor made arrangements for the family to take Brennan to the hospital in Richmond, about an hour from her home. She called her parents, and her stepfather took

Brennan's twin brother, Patrick, home. Her mother then drove Kearsten and Brennan to the hospital.

On the way there, Kearsten was in shock. She knew diabetes was something terrible. Her ex-husband hadn't taken care of himself, and he was already suffering from health problems at the age of 28. She blamed herself because she knew that the disease was genetic, and she had had children with a man who was diabetic. She had always known it was a possibility, but she was hoping it wouldn't happen to either of her babies. Kearsten kept thinking, "How could God do this to my beautiful baby? How will I be able to cope with taking care of a diabetic?"

Brennan was checked into the hospital where he was immediately given a shot of insulin. Because he was so young, he stayed in a tall crib with bars that reminded Kearsten of a jail cell. Sometimes she lowered the side rail and crawled into the crib just to hold him and stay close to him. She stayed with him that night and every night for 4 days. It was hard to accept that he had this diagnosis when he seemed okay. During his stay, he flirted with the nurses and had the run of the halls. But Kearsten roamed those same halls and saw the really sick babies, and she accepted the truth.

On the second day, Kearsten gave Brennan his shot. The nurses kept saying the shot would go in very easily, but it was one of the hardest things his mother had ever done, and she knew eventually he would have to do it every day, and for the rest of his life. While in the hospital, Kearsten met with dieticians, nurses, and doctors. She learned Brennan's eating habits would not have to change too much, as she had always tried to serve nutritious meals. She also learned how to test Brennan's blood, where to give him shots, and what to do if his blood sugars went too high or too low. Brennan's father and his family also came to visit Brennan in the hospital. His father cried, as he also blamed himself for Brennan having diabetes. Even though Kearsten knew it was really no one's fault, it was still hard to be kind to him because she was so angry.

After the 4 days in the hospital Kearsten's family came to get her and Brennan. They were making the trip home, and Brennan's blood sugar was better, but Kearsten knew this was only the beginning of a very long, difficult journey. She kept thinking of what her ex-husband's mother had once told her. She said, "It's so hard to know your child may die before you." Now Kearsten had those same thoughts about her own precious son. How was she going to handle the day-to-day challenges of having a child with diabetes? Kearsten also had a special challenge; how was she going deal with her son as a twin? Brennan had diabetes, but Patrick did not. How was she going to be fair while still accepting the fact that her two children had very different needs?

The day parents discover their child has diabetes is one of the worst days of their lives. All sorts of question, fears, and doubts come to mind. Will he or she be okay? Will I be able to give shots? How much does it hurt to test blood? What changes do I have to make to his or her diet? Will my child be able to enjoy holidays like Halloween and Easter? What will I even do about birthday cakes? And HOW WILL I MANAGE IT ALL? Being a parent of diabetic child is a challenge at any age, but each stage has special needs that parents must understand.

AGES AND STAGES

Baby/Toddler Years

Parents of very young children with diabetes deal with one of the most difficult challenges. Nurses need to alert parents that young children lack the ability to communicate how they feel. For example, sometimes it is even difficult to be aware the child is showing symptoms of diabetes. A parent may not be aware his or her child's overly wet diaper or constant drinking is a sign of diabetes, unless that parent is already familiar with the signs. Frequently, a baby or toddler must be pretty sick in order for the parent to take the child to the doctor.

Once diagnosed and sent home from the hospital, parents must not only learn how to initially treat the disease; they must also become *detectives* when trying to determine how the child is feeling. "Is my child showing signs of low blood sugar? Is he or she acting 'high'?" It is very difficult to figure this out when the child is unable to use words to communicate with his or her parent. Many parents of babies, toddlers, and preschoolers are in constant contact with their nurses and physicians, simply because they can't tell. Parents should keep a log of questions they have and call the nurse weekly for answers and clarification.

Nurses should remind parents that they know their child better than anyone. For example, one child may cry uncontrollably over something he or she would never cry about, and this could mean the child is "low."

Other children may become sleepy or cranky or even angry. Still others will show signs of low blood sugar physically rather than emotionally. They may appear shaky or unstable. Maybe it's a look in the child's eyes that only the parents understand. Parents must have more faith in their ability to know that something is wrong and use these clues to figure out what it is. This is difficult because their child was just diagnosed with something new and scary. To parents, it feels like they are bringing home that tiny newborn baby all over again.

At the point a child is diagnosed, it is important for nurses to assess parent expectations of their health care professional. Get to know their personality. Some parents may want exact instructions while others may need the freedom to experiment with what works for their child. Attention to these details will put parents more at ease, making the transition to diabetes management easier for the patient, the child's parents, and the whole family.

Parents must become familiar with the signs of low and high blood sugars in general and then determine what applies specifically to their child. See Table 8.1 for signs and symptoms of hypo- and hyperglycemia in a young child.

The School-Age Child

In this stage, it is very important for all parents to remember they have rights within the school system. Whether entering school with a child who has been previously diagnosed with diabetes or whether a child who has been in school has been recently diagnosed, schools are responsible for the care of the child enrolled. This is the law!

For those children entering school with diabetes, it is imperative for parents to inform the school beforehand and meet with the professionals in charge of the child's care. This includes the school nurse, the regular education teacher, the physical education teacher, and any other educational professional deemed necessary by the parents and school. At this time, a plan will be devised to most effectively manage the child's diabetes (ADA, 2006, p. S49). There are three basic types of plans within the schools.

Diabetes Medical Management Plan (DMMP)

The Diabetes Medical Management Plan is a plan that includes information on who is responsible for diabetes management, instructions on how

TABLE 8.1 Signs and Symptoms of Hypoglycemia and Hyperglycemia in Children

Hypoglycemia	Young child	Hyperglycemia	Young child
Tremors, shakiness, jerky movements	Same	Excessive urination	Soaked diapers or accidents if potty trained
Dizziness, feeling faint, headache	Lethargic, unable to sit up	Excessive thirst	Crying for more fluids
		Excessive hunger	Craving sweets
Sweating, pale moist skin	Same	Headache	Crying more than usual
Excessive hunger	Craving sweets	Sleepiness	Sleeping longer than usual
Mood swings or erratic behavior	Irritability	Difficulty concentrating	Not able to do usual tasks
Tingling or numbness	Difficult to assess	Visual disturbances	Difficulty focusing
Difficulty paying attention, confusion	Same	Dry or flushed skin	Same
Visual disturbances, dilated pupils	Dilated pupils	General malaise	Crying without relief, irritable
Increased heart and respiratory rates	Same	Weight loss	Same
		Fruity breath	Same, sweet odor to urine
Seizures and coma	Same	Coma	Same

to handle emergency situations, specific instructions for how to deal with levels of high and low blood sugars, and basic "rules of thumb" on how to deal with the child's needs. For example, one parent might wish to be called if the blood sugar is lower than 70. However, another child's DMMP may state to simply give the child a snack and check blood sugar in 15 minutes.

See Table 8.2 for content that should be on a DMMP. Quite often, the DMMP is all that is required to make sure the child's diabetic needs are being met (Lawlor & Pasquarello, 2004). A parent who is interested in obtaining a DMMP should call the American Diabetes Association at 1-800-DIABETES (342-3837).

504 Plan

A 504 Plan is used if a parent either does not feel the child's needs are being met with the DMMP or the parent feels the child is being discriminated against due to his or her diabetes. For example, a child who is not allowed to eat a snack in the classroom may miss valuable class time leaving to eat, and consequently, the child's grades may suffer.

Section 504 of the Rehabilitation Act of 1973 is a civil rights law that prohibits disability-based discrimination in all programs that receive or benefit from federal financial assistance. A 504 Plan is a legal agreement between the student and a school to ensure the child will be able to participate in all activities while having his or her diabetic needs met. If a parent wishes for a 504 Plan to be put in place, the parents first contact the guidance department of their child's school. At that time, a team will meet to determine if a 504 Plan is necessary. The team usually consists of the parent(s), guidance counselor, regular education teacher, school nurse, and other necessary school personnel. It is important for parents to remember they have the right to a 504 Plan if they feel it is necessary to avoid any discrimination due to diabetes. A 504 Plan may include many of the guidelines put in place by the DMMP; however, a 504 Plan is a legal document, and the school must comply with it by law (ADA, n.d.).

Individualized Education Plan (IEP)

An Individualized Education Plan is for those diabetic students who have special educational needs that affect the child's academic performance. Many children with diabetes who have an IEP are labeled as Other Health Impaired (OHI). This means that diabetic-related complications significantly affect the child's ability to learn. For example, a child with extremely fluctuating blood sugars may have difficulty paying attention in class, which in turn would affect his or her ability to learn. With an IEP, accommodations such as extra time on assignments or repeating of directions will be put into place to help improve the child's performance.

TABLE 8.2   What Should be Included in a DMMP

Diabetes management	Insulin	Meal planning
Who performs the blood glucose test?	What type(s) of insulin does the student take?	What time does the student eat lunch?
What type of meter is used?	Where is the insulin stored?	Does he or she eat a school lunch or bring lunch from home?
Where is the meter stored and used?		Is there a plan if the student refuses to eat lunch?
Who writes down monitoring results and where?		
How should parents be informed of blood glucose results and treatments?	How is the insulin stored?	Who is responsible for making sure the student eats a snack?
What are the blood glucose target ranges?	How is the insulin dose determined?	Does the school restrict where food can be eaten?
What action is to be taken if the blood glucose level is outside the target range?	When is insulin administered?	Can snacks be eaten in the classroom?
Are ketones to be checked?	Who administers insulin?	If the whole class has a snack, how will the student with diabetes be accommodated?
At what blood glucose level should ketones be checked?		Are there classroom parties or special projects that involve food?
By whom should they be checked?		If so, what are the guidelines and accommodations for the student with diabetes?
What should be done with information on ketones?		

Putting an IEP into place is a process that takes some time. Usually, a child must be referred for an initial meeting. Those present usually include the same team as that needed for a 504 Plan, in addition to a school social worker and a school psychologist. Several components are then needed to determine if the child is eligible for an IEP. These may include a medical history and exam, interview of the family by the school social worker, teacher evaluations, classroom observations, and various diagnostic tests given by the school psychologist. The team will then reconvene to determine the significance of the data. If a significant discrepancy is found between learning ability and achievement, then the child will qualify for an IEP.

The IEP will include goals to improve the child's educational performance. Within these goals accommodations will be created. The DMMP serves as a good basis for the goals. An IEP is a legal document that must be reviewed once a year. The parents also have the right to review the goals and make changes at any time if they are not pleased with their child's performance or the plan is not meeting the child's needs.

The DMMP, 504 Plan, and IEP are all plans designed to ensure the best care for a child with diabetes. It is the right of the parents to decide which plan(s) is (are) the best for their child.

The Prepubescent Child

As if diabetes were not enough of a challenge itself, children between the ages of 9 and 12 have a whole new set of challenges. After all, they are about to become teenagers!

For those children age 9–12 who have been diabetic for some time, parents are frequently lulled into thinking their child is capable of taking on his or her own diabetic care. The nurse should remind parents that while most children are capable of performing the daily medical tasks, they are not emotionally ready to assume all the responsibility for their care. For example, almost all diabetic children at this age are able to test their own blood and even give themselves an injection. However, a 9-year-old probably will not be able to correctly measure the insulin for the syringe, especially if half units are necessary. Children in this age group are also not able to comprehend how serious it is to measure the appropriate amount and the consequences of giving themselves too much or too little insulin.

The prepubescent child is also prone to "cheating" or "sneaking," as it is sometimes called. This is the age of peer pressure, and many children want to be "normal" and eat junk and sugary foods. Parents must be mindful of cheating, and nurses should advise them to keep a close eye on their child's blood sugar levels, but it must be handled while still respecting the growing independence of their child. Some parents allow their child to test his or her blood, but the parents record the readings. By doing this, parents can see if there are highs at certain times. If so, then the child should be asked what might have caused the high reading. If high blood sugars become a pattern, then parents must work to find the underlying cause (Schmidt, 2003).

For example, a child consistently has high blood sugar readings at dinner. After some discussion, the parents find that their child walks home with a group of children who like to buy extra pies and candy at lunch in order to have something to eat on the way home from school. When offered the snacks, she eats them because she is too embarrassed to tell her friends she is diabetic and can't eat them. This results in an extremely high blood sugar at dinner.

What should a parent do in this situation? First, parents must remember their child is human, and all people, including parents themselves, eat food they should not. No one is perfect at all times, and children are desperate to fit in with their peers. It is important not to blame the child. Once the child is caught, he or she usually feels badly enough without adding on extra guilt. The best approach is to sit down with the child and talk about why the child cheated. Find out the underlying cause of the cheating and acknowledge it. If it is due to peer pressure, parents must be empathetic and explain that they understand the importance of fitting in with friends. In the case of peer pressure, parents must continually remind their child of the importance of keeping blood sugars under control in order to best take care of his or her body. Perhaps the child is going through a growth spurt and is seriously hungry at that time of day. If so, then parents should work with the child to incorporate an appropriate snack into his or her meal plan so that cheating is no longer necessary.

Sometimes children at this age are starting to rebel against the fact that they have diabetes. They become angry with their situation and decide to ignore the consequences of not taking care of themselves properly. Parents may need to enlist the support of someone outside the family, such as a teacher, nurse, guidance counselor, or coach, to provide positive support to the child. These people may be able to gently steer the child back on to a more rigorous management plan for his or her diabetes. It is important for parents to remember that these behaviors are normal for their child's age and that diabetes is simply another area that will involve the normal growing pains of independence and questioning of authority.

There are many resources for teachers, child care providers, parents, and health professionals. For a comprehensive list and directions for obtaining copies, call the American Diabetes Association at 1-800-DIABETES (342-3837).

REFERENCES

American Diabetes Association. (n.d.). *Your school and your rights.* Retrieved January 8, 2006, from http://www.diabetes.org/advocacy-and-legalresources/discrimination/school/scrights.jsp

American Diabetes Association. (2006). Diabetes care in school and day care settings. *Diabetes Care. 29,* S49–S55.

Lawlor, M. T., & Pasquarello, C. (2004, May/June). School planning 101. *Diabetes Self-Management*, pp. 69–74.

Schmidt, C. (2003, November/December). Mothers' perceptions of self-care in school-age children with diabetes. *MCN, 28*(6), 363–370.

9

Adolescents With Diabetes

Beverly Baliko

Nobody can make you feel inferior without your consent.

Eleanor Roosevelt

The expected developmental struggles and transitions of adolescent life are complicated by the necessity of managing diabetes. The type of diabetes, as well as many other factors, has a role in determining the best approach to care. New issues may arise when adolescents with type 1 diabetes, though accustomed to living with the disease, begin to assert their independence and seek more autonomy in self-management. The onset of type 2 diabetes, however, can present even more complex challenges. The nurse is in a position to advocate for both adolescents and their families in the quest to achieve optimal wellness and prepare for lifelong management of this chronic condition.

Adolescence is a time of rapid physiological, cognitive, psychological, and social change that also requires adaptation within the family system. Physiologically, the onset of puberty is accompanied by dramatic hormonal shifts that drive the obvious physical changes, as well as the often intense and unpredictable fluctuations in mood that characterize the teen years. Cognitively, adolescents begin to develop new problem-solving skills, think more abstractly, and test previous assumptions about the world. They begin to develop a personal sense of morality and values and attempt to define and express their identity as individuals. Although they can visualize and plan for the future, many adolescents tend to be quite present-oriented, with little consideration for long-term consequences of their behaviors. Impulsivity and a sense of invulnerability may contribute to a willingness to take risks. Increasing importance is placed on self-image, sexuality, and peer acceptance. Family relationships are being redefined and boundaries renegotiated.

What do these changes mean in terms of diabetes management? First, the physiological changes associated with adolescence lead to blood glucose fluctuations and insulin resistance, making glycemic control in this population more difficult to achieve. Unfortunately, other manifestations of adolescent development can interact to further complicate matters. The desire to be spontaneous, conform to social norms, and avoid appearing different can lead some adolescents, especially younger ones, to take risks with their health (Muscari, 1998; Scheiner, Brow, & Phillips, 2000). The normative developmental movement toward independence and individuality that contributes to parent-teen conflicts in general may be enacted in various aspects of diabetes management. Teenagers may want increased responsibility and control in managing their condition and resent the degree of dependence on parents and health care professions that is necessary to help ensure their ongoing wellness (Scheiner et al., 2000). The response to perceived interference may be rebellion against regimented treatment protocols. As a group, adolescents are already predisposed to the development of depression and anxiety. Coping with the demands of a chronic illness such as diabetes can further tax teenagers' emotional resources and the resources of the family as a system.

BALANCING PARENTAL INVOLVEMENT

Despite the desire for autonomy, adolescents both need and want parental involvement in their diabetes care. Studies have indicated a correlation between family conflict, adherence problems, and poorer glucose control and improved glucose control with a team approach to parental involvement (Anderson, Bracket, Ho, & Laffel, 1999; Miller-Johnson et al., 1994). The challenge is to find the line between too much involvement and too little. Many years ago, Coyne, Wortman, and Lehman (1988) used the term "miscarried helping" for excessive parental attempts to provide care that undermined healthy adolescent development. Attempts to coerce adolescents to comply typically result in resistance. Other adolescents, especially those who are newly diagnosed with diabetes, might be overwhelmed and regress to earlier developmental levels. Parents who are too attentive or overprotective concerning their child's illness can unknowingly reinforce excessively dependent behaviors. On the other hand, parental expectations that the adolescent will assume too much responsibility too quickly also result in poor outcomes

(Wysocki et al., 1996). Weissberg-Benchell and Antisdel (2000) concluded that the transfer of responsibility for carrying out tasks related to the management of diabetes should occur gradually, with continued parental involvement throughout the process.

Working individually with adolescents, in addition to working with them within the family setting, helps build trust and demonstrates respect for the teenager's desire for independence. Teaching adolescents coping skills related to managing stress, setting priorities, and problem solving in potentially awkward social situations can help prepare teenagers to assume greater responsibility in their self-care (Scheiner et al., 2000). Successful use of such skills is reassuring to both adolescents and their parents as new roles are being negotiated.

Parents of adolescents who have been helping their child to manage their diabetes for many years may need help determining how much control to relinquish and when the adolescent is developmentally ready to assume more autonomy. It is important for the caregiver not to assume that parents will require little support or education. Coping with an adolescent is challenging for parents; coping with an adolescent with diabetes can be much more challenging. Parents of newly diagnosed adolescents will need education concerning their child's condition and its management. This is a good opportunity for nurses to help foster an atmosphere of cooperation and closeness between parents and adolescents as they face the new situation together.

NONADHERENCE IN ADOLESCENTS WITH DIABETES

Even teenagers with type 1 diabetes who are knowledgeable about their condition and have been previously compliant with treatment regimens may exhibit sudden shifts in attitude and behavior that are a cause of alarm to parents and caregivers. Responding with rigidity and confrontation is likely to be met with hostility and conflict. Adolescents, struggling toward independence, may rebel against parents and health care providers who they perceive to be authority figures. However, allowing adolescents to assume full responsibility for their diabetes management too soon can be risky, too. Either response can result in nonadherence.

Rebellion is not the only contributor to adolescent nonadherence to diabetes regimens. Because teenagers are at different points in their development of abstract thinking skills, they may genuinely not comprehend the long-term consequences of nonadherence. Some adolescents respond to a concern about self-concept and body image by attempting to avoid an appearance of being different from their peers.

The first step toward intervening in teenage nonadherence is understanding what concerns drive the teenager's behavior. Attempt to rule out underlying problems such as depression, eating disorders, and substance abuse that may affect motivation, cognition, mood, and actions. Depression is a common problem during adolescence. The additional stressor of coping with a chronic illness can heighten a preexisting risk. Although eating disorders can occur at any time in life, because of adolescent preoccupation with appearance and susceptibility to media ideals, adolescence is the most frequent stage at which they develop. There is some evidence to suggest that eating disorders occur more frequently in adolescents with diabetes then in the general population (Daneman, 2002). Other studies have indicated that between 15% and 39% of young women with diabetes manipulate their insulin with a goal of weight control (Biggs, Basco, Patterson, & Raskin, 1994; Peveler, Fairburn, Boller, & Donger, 1992; Polonsky et al., 1994). Adolescents may do this without awareness of or concern for the damage it is doing to their bodies. Binging and purging can cause dangerous fluctuations in blood glucose. Eating disorders are associated with poorer glycemic control and with long-term complications (Affenito et al., 1997; Rydall, Rodin, Olmsted, Devenyi, & Daneman, 1997). Vomiting after binging on food or alcohol can lead to ketoacidosis. If you suspect that an adolescent with whom you are working is depressed, abusing substances, or has an eating disorder, refer the adolescent for counseling. You can work collaboratively with mental health professionals to help ensure that the adolescent receives comprehensive care that addresses emotional and physiological needs.

Most often, nonadherence is a behavioral response associated with adolescent development. It is especially important to foster a trusting relationship with adolescents who have diabetes. Being empathetic to their concerns, taking time to listen, maintaining confidentiality, providing positive reinforcement for healthy behaviors, and including them as collaborators in their treatment planning will help achieve this goal. Muscari (1998) suggests working with your adolescent client to create a formal contract. The written contract should outline the desired outcome and the interventions required to achieve it. Because adolescents live in the present, setting short-term, realistic goals will be more effective than focusing on long-term consequences.

While you must tailor your interactions and teaching to each individual's cognitive level, avoid talking down to adolescent clients, and treat them as individuals who are capable of making healthy choices. These approaches will help counteract the tendency for adolescents to rebel in order to assert their own identity. Working collaboratively will permit a sense of control and increase your chances of gaining your adolescent client's cooperation.

Many adolescents lead busy lives and have full schedules. If some adolescents perceive diabetes self-management to be too time-consuming or inconvenient, you can work with the clients to help incorporate their therapeutic regimens into their daily routines, making interventions less disruptive. Teenagers value flexibility and spontaneity. Attempts to ban specific foods or strictly regulate activities are likely to be unsuccessful. Instead, teach teenagers how to make reasonable food choices and adjust their medication to accommodate what they eat. It may be time to think about modifying the adolescent's medication or consider use of a pump.

When teaching, use instructional methods that that will stimulate and hold your clients' interest. Most teenagers are frequent and competent users of the Internet. You can direct them to Web sites where they will find accurate information about their illness (see the list at the end of this chapter). Online discussion groups can be a means of both information and peer support. Parents may find the Internet a valuable resource as well. Because teenagers value peer acceptance and interaction, support groups and camps can provide them with a peer group who shares their health challenges. Reid, Dubow, Carey, and Dura (1994) found that teenagers who adhered to their diabetes treatment regimen tended to actively seek social support and use problem-solving techniques to cope with their illness. Check local hospitals, clinics, pediatricians' offices, or newspapers to find resources in your area for children with diabetes and their families. The Diabetes Education and Camping Association has a listing of camping opportunities available at http://www.diabetescamps. org. Of note: Although many adolescents find support groups and camping experiences to be normalizing, others may perceive them as emphasizing their differences. If so, avoid pushing the adolescent to participate.

A collaborative, validating approach, creativity and flexibility in care planning, and acknowledgment of the adolescent's need for support are strategies that can potentially decrease the problem of nonadherence in adolescents with diabetes. Above all, genuinely attempt to achieve an understanding of the adolescent's perspective on his or her illness.

What does having diabetes mean to adolescents? What do they believe about long-term consequences? How do they think having diabetes affects them personally and socially? What are their priorities in life? What problems do they anticipate in managing their diabetes? Stepping into the adolescent's world will help you, the nurse, to be viewed as a partner, rather than an adversary, in helping the adolescent to achieve optimal wellness.

REFERENCES

Affenito, S. G., Backstrand, J. R., Welch, G. W., Lammi-Keefe, C. J., Rodriguez, N. R., & Adams, C. H. (1997). Subclinical and clinical eating disorders in IDDM negatively affect metabolic control. *Diabetes Care, 20,* 183–184.

Anderson, B. J., Bracket, J., Ho, J., & Laffel, L. M. B. (1999). An office-based intervention to maintain parent-adolescent teamwork in diabetes management: Impact on parent involvement, family conflict, subsequent glycolic control. *Diabetes Care, 22,* 713–721.

Biggs, M. M., Basco, M. R., Patterson, G., & Raskin, P. (1994). Insulin withholding for weight control in women with diabetes. *Diabetes Care, 17,* 1186–1189.

Coyne, J., Wortman, C., & Lehman, D. (1988). The other side of support: Emotional overinvolvement and miscarried helping. In B. Botlieb (Ed.), *Social support: Formats, processes, and effects* (pp. 305–333). New York: Sage.

Daneman, D. (2002). Eating disorders in adolescent girls and young women with type 1 diabetes. *Diabetes Spectrum, 15,* 83–105.

Miller-Johnson, S., Emery, R. E., Marvin, R. S., Clarke, W., Lovinger, R., & Martin, M. (1994). Parent-child relationships and the management of insulin-dependent diabetes mellitus. *Journal of Consulting and Clinical Psychology, 62,* 603–610.

Muscari, M. E. (1998). Rebels with a cause: When adolescents won't follow medical advice. *American Journal of Nursing, 98,* 26–30.

Peveler, R. C., Fairburn, C. G., Boller, I., & Donger, D. (1992). Eating disorders in adolescents with IDDM: A controlled study. *Diabetes Care, 15,* 1356–1360.

Polonsky, W. H., Anderson, B. J., Lohrer, P. A., Apente, J. E., Jacobson, A. M., & Cole, C. F. (1994). Insulin omission in women with IDDM. *Diabetes Care, 17,* 1178–1185.

Reid, G. J., Dubow, E. F., Carey, T. C., & Dura, J. R. (1994). Contribution of coping to medical adjustment and treatment responsibility among children and adolescents with diabetes. *Journal of Developmental and Behavioral Pediatrics, 14,* 327–335.

Rydall, A. C., Rodin, G. M., Olmsted, M. P., Devenyi, R. G., & Daneman, D. (1997). Disordered eating behavior and microvascular complications in young women with insulin-dependent diabetes mellitus. *New England Journal of Medicine, 336,* 1849–1854.

Scheiner, B., Brow, S., & Phillips, M. (2000). Management strategies for the adolescent lifestyle. *Diabetes Spectrum, 13,* 83–88.

Weissberg-Benchell, J., & Antisdel, J. E. (2000). Balancing developmental needs and intensive management in adolescents. *Diabetes Spectrum, 13,* 88–94.

Wysocki, T., Taylor, A., Hough, B. S., Linscheid, T. R., Yeates, K. O., & Naglieri, J. A. (1996). Deviation from developmentally appropriate self-care autonomy. *Diabetes Care, 19,* 199–125.

ONLINE RESOURCES

American Diabetes Association, http://www.diabetes.org/for-parents-and-kids/for-teens.jsp

Children with Diabetes, http://www.childrenwithdiabetes.com

Juvenile Diabetes Research Foundational International, http://www.jdrf.org

National Diabetes Education Program, http://www.ndep.nih.gov/diabetes/youth/youth.htm

10

Diabetes in Adults With Special Needs

There is only one way ... to get anybody to do anything. And that is by making the other person want to do it.

Dale Carnegie

Most of chapter 7, "The Nurse as Teacher," could apply to many adult clients, but there are two groups of adults with diabetes who are particularly vulnerable to accelerating tissue damage and, perhaps, more amenable to intervention. In my view, these include pregnant women and the aging population.

DIABETES AND PREGNANCY

Pregestational Diabetes

Many women often wonder about the effects of pregnancy on their body, but women with preexisting diabetes have good reason to be concerned.

Type 1 Diabetes

Years ago women with type 1 diabetes diagnosed as children were discouraged from getting pregnant. Prior to the development of insulin in 1922, children with diabetes did not live long enough to procreate. Anyone who remembers seeing the 1989 film *Steel Magnolias* is aware that pregnancy can cause damage to glucose-sensitive organs in women with type 1 diabetes. In the film, Julia Roberts plays a type 1 childhood diabetic. She is warned not to attempt pregnancy by her physician and her mother. She does so anyway, has a difficult time with the pregnancy and delivery, and ends up dying of renal failure a year later. Even though there have been y advances made in the care of pregnant women in general, and those with diabetes in particular, many parents of young diabetic women may still consider pregnancy a death sentence for their daughters. More sophisticated glucose meters, rapid-acting insulin, insulin pumps, and research have greatly impacted the safety of pregnancy for women with diabetes. More women with long-standing disease have fewer complications today due to better glycemic control before pregnancy, decreasing potential complications.

Pregnancy for anyone is considered a complex metabolic state causing dramatic shifts in glucose, fat, and protein utilization. During the first trimester, the body is insulin sensitive and burns more fat for energy than usual, thus decreasing insulin demands. Many women are also nauseated and normal weight gain is typically less than 4 pounds during this time. Some women actually lose weight due to nausea and vomiting. As the placenta becomes fully functional during the second trimester, it produces increasing amount of hormones (human placental growth hormone, human placental lactogen, and progesterose) that cause insulin resistance. By the third trimester, the pancreas must produce up to three times the amount of insulin for the body to remain euglycemic. In addition, the basal metabolic rate increases tremendously and both the woman's demands for glucose and that of her fetus are considerable. Normally, weight gain during the second and third trimester equals up to a pound per week with a total weight gain of 25–35 pounds. During normal pregnancy, women have a lower fasting glucose and are hyperinsulinemic due to the increase in glucose uptake by the fetoplacental unit and by the cells of their own bodies. With a normal pancreas, the added insulin needs are fulfilled automatically. When an actual diabetic state is added to the normal changes in pregnancy, glycemic control is further challenged. The consequences of not controlling blood sugars to the pregnant woman can include a worsening of any preexisting long-term complications, such as retinopathy, nephropathy, neuropathy, hypertension, and cardiovascular disease. Even without preexisting diabetic complications, these women are at increased risk for pregnancy-inducted hypertension (PIH), miscarriage, and diabetic ketoacidosis (DKA), as well as the beginning of chronic long-term complications, if glycemic control is not achieved. Preconception care for women with diabetes to achieve blood sugar control is also important to prevent miscarriages and congenital anomalies. Maternal hyperglycemia can be teratogenic in the first few weeks of gestation when organogenesis is taking place. The resulting birth defects most often include neural tube defects and cardiac anomalies, as well as those of skeletal, renal, genitourinary, and gastrointestinal systems, and chromosomal anomalies (Barss & Repke, 2005). With uncontrolled glucose levels later on in pregnancy, the fetus grows larger than normal (macrosomia), making vaginal birth difficult or impossible. This increases the likelihood of shoulder dystocia, fractured clavicle, or the need for a cesarean delivery. Hyperglycemia also increases the stillbirth and perinatal mortality rates. The infant of a diabetic mother with uncontrolled blood sugars is at risk for jaundice, respiratory distress syndrome (especially if macrosomic), and prematurity. Macrosomic babies usually have more fat cells than normal and are at risk for obesity and type 2 diabetes during their lifetime.

Type 2 Diabetes

Women with pregestational type 2 diabetes are often overweight and may have hypertension. It is as important for these women to prepare for pregnancy as it is for women with type 1 diabetes. A study conducted by Clausen et al. comparing women with type 2 diabetes to women with type 1 diabetes and those without diabetes concluded that perinatal mortality increased by four to nine times and major congenital anomalies were more than doubled in women with type 2 diabetes. Type 2 diabetes is a lot more than just a touch of sugar. The women in this study were older, overweight, had more children and were often non-White, with a shorter duration of time since diagnosis and had A1Cs during pregnancy that were lower than women with type 1 diabetes. This seems to be counterintuitive. However, most clients with type 1 diabetes were in better glycemic control before pregnancy, planned the pregnancy, sought prenatal care earlier, were of normal weight, and were younger with fewer pregnancies than those with type 2 diabetes. Many of the women with type 2 diabetes had metabolic syndrome and were insulin resistant prior to pregnancy. This study points out the importance of having women with type 2 diabetes prepare their bodies for pregnancy by losing weight, controlling blood pressure, and controlling blood sugars, often with insulin, because most oral agents are teratogenic in the first trimester (Clausen et al., 2005). Glyburide, a sulfonylurea, has been given after 24 weeks of gestation and shown not to cross the placenta or cause any fetal problems. This might be a good choice for treatment of gestational diabetes, which develops about this time.

Metformin (Glucophage) can be used in the first trimester for women with polycystic ovarian disease to reverse infertility and prevent early miscarriage; however, there is an increased risk of preeclampsia, and because this drug does cross the placenta, there is an increased risk of fetal anomalies (Barbour & Friedman, 2003).

Gestational Diabetes

Gestational diabetes mellitus (GDM) is diagnosed only during the later half of pregnancy. Blood sugars usually return to normal after delivery of the placenta. The above-mentioned placental hormones cause increasing insulin resistance as the pregnancy progresses and may outpace the pancreas's ability to increase insulin production in some women. The screening tool for gestational diabetes given to pregnant women between 24–28 weeks consists of a glucose challenge test. A 50-gram Glucola solution is administered orally, and a serum glucose is obtained 1 hour later. A blood sugar greater than 130 mg/dl will identify around 90% of women who have gestational diabetes (Barbour & Friedman, 2003). This subset of women should then receive a 3-hour, 100-gram oral glucose tolerance test (OGTT). See Table 10.1 for criteria for a positive OGTT. Meeting or exceeding any two values is regarded as a positive test and is diagnostic of gestational diabetes. If only one value is met or exceeded, a repeat 3-hour OGTT is scheduled 1 month later. The American Diabetes Association (ADA, 2006, p. S7) recommends testing all pregnant women at 24–28 weeks of gestation who fall into the following risk categories:

1. older than 24 years
2. overweight or obese with a BMI greater than 25
3. history of poor obstetrical outcome or an infant considered large for gestational age
4. GDM diagnosed in a previous pregnancy
5. diagnosis of prediabetes
6. first-degree relatives with type 2 diabetes
7. ancestry from high risk population (African American, Asian American, Native American Indians, Mexican American, and Pacific Islanders such as Hawaiians and Filipinos)

Anyone who does not fall into one of these categories need not be tested (ADA, 2006, p. S7). Gestational diabetes represents 90% of all pregnancies complicated by diabetes. About 135,000 cases are diagnosed each year, equaling 4% of all pregnancies in the United States. With the obesity rates of women in their childbearing years (15–44) increasing, the rate of gestational diabetes should also increase in the near future. This diagnosis increases the risk for these women of being diagnosed with type 2 diabetes often within 5–10 years of the pregnancy (ADA, n.d.). Three abnormalities make glucose regulation during pregnancy more difficult than normal for women diagnosed with gestational diabetes (GDM): (1) insulin resistance is common for the third trimester for all women; (2) however, glucose metabolism of women with GDM is further hampered by impaired insulin secretion; and (3) increased hepatic glucose production. Their insulin resistance is greater than in normal pregnancies during the third trimester, thus compounding the problem, resulting in hyperglycemia.

Teaching and Motivating Pregnant Clients

The above information gives the nurse abundant ammunition to motivate women with diabetes to control blood sugars before and during pregnancy. Following hb A1C levels every 3 months will evaluate the success of their efforts and indicate when attempting pregnancy is optimal. Women who are not seen regularly are more likely to become pregnant without the benefit of good glycemic control and may well develop some of the complications discussed above. When most women plan a pregnancy, they are excited and eager to have a healthy, uncomplicated pregnancy and birth. They are motivated to eat a healthy diet, get some exercise, and follow advice given. This may be the most optimal time to teach women with diabetes good glycemic control.

Blood sugar ranges during pregnancy are the same for diabetic and nondiabetic women, a point that should make a woman with diabetes feel normal perhaps for the first time since her diagnosis. These ranges (see Table 10.1) are about 20% lower than for those who are not pregnant and are easy to achieve in nondiabetic women because their needed increase in insulin is automatic. Those who cannot overcome the pregnancy-induced insulin resistance by producing more and more insulin as the pregnancy progresses develop gestational diabetes. Because gestational diabetes

TABLE 10.1   Diagnostic Criteria for Gestational Diabetes

Using 100-gram, 3-hour Oral Glucose Tolerance Test (OGTT) two or more of the following values must be met:

Fasting	≥ 95 mg/dl
1 hour	≥ 180 mg/dl
2 hours	≥ 155 mg/dl
3 hours	≥ 140 mg/dl

Note. From "Standards of Medical Care in Diabetics 2006," *Diabetes Care, 29,* S7. Copyright © 2006 by the American Diabetes Association. Modified with permission from the American Diabetes Association.

increases their risk for complications during pregnancy and the risk of a large baby complicating delivery, these women should also be acutely interested in learning how to control blood sugars. The following list of topics should be covered with anyone with pregestational or gestational diabetes. It should be stressed that these are areas of concern for general diabetic care and good glycemic control and should be continued after pregnancy as well.

1. Home glucose monitoring should be done at least before meals and at bedtime. Women with type 2 diabetes and gestational diabetes should periodically test 2 hours after a meal. Following 2-hour postprandial blood sugar will indicate whether or not appropriate steps are being taken to control glucose spikes because this is most strongly correlated with fetal macrosomia. See Table 10.1 for normal ranges.

2. A dietician may be needed to review current eating habits and make appropriate recommendations for change as needed. Diets that do not accommodate a client's likes and dislikes or her financial constraints are a waste of time and effort. Individualizing a diet to meet the nutritional requirements of pregnancy is paramount. Decreasing carbohydrates to 45% of total calories may be necessary to blunt postprandial blood sugars for women with type 2 and gestational diabetes. For obese women, it might be necessary to decrease not only carbohydrate intake but total amount of calories as well. A caloric intake of 2,200 kcal (an expected increase of 300 calories for most women) might be a drastic reduction for those with type 2 or gestational diabetes. However, this caloric amount should achieve a

weight gain of around 15 pounds for those who are obese, resulting in a normal size baby and weight loss for the woman during post-partum. A diet low in fat, moderate in animal protein, and high in whole grains and fiber with five to nine servings of fresh fruit and vegetables and four servings of low-fat dairy should meet the needs of pregnancy.

3. Moderate exercise is recommended for all pregnant women. It is particularly important to help maintain glycemic control in women with diabetes. The concern for anyone pregnant is to avoid exceeding a heart rate of 150 beats per minute lasting no more than 1 hour. Prevention of dehydration and heat exhaustion is important, for these conditions affect the baby as well. Low-impact aerobic, weight-bearing exercise three times per week should greatly enhance a feeling of well being. Nurses should help women to make time for exercise. Anyone on insulin should be cautioned to exercise after eating or to test blood sugar to prevent hypoglycemia.

4. Insulin does not cross the placenta and is the drug of choice for both type 1 and type 2 clients during pregnancy. Type 2 diabetics on oral hypoglycemic agents should expect to be switched to insulin prior to pregnancy. If they are on antihypertensives, especially ACE inhibitors and angiotensin receptor blockers (ARBs), they need to know that other medication will be substituted because these drugs are particularly teratogenic. The literature supports use of older antihypertensives, such as methyldopa (Aldomet), hydralazine (Apresoline), and nifedipine (Procardia), during pregnancy. Women diagnosed with gestational diabetes may be able to control blood sugars with diet and exercise or may need medication such as glyburide or insulin after 24 weeks.

The nurse's role in helping these women understand how diabetes affects their pregnancy, delivery, and newborn is invaluable. Listening to their real concerns and working with them will help ensure their compliance with instructions. They may be some of the most motivated clients with whom the nurse has ever worked. In reviewing the learning principles used in chapter 7 and listed in Table 7.2, this population is usually eager to learn; willing to increase their knowledge of glycemic control; usually interested in having a healthy pregnancy, easy delivery, and healthy baby; and willing to learn or relearn how to do blood sugars and actively participate in the decision making that results. If the client is new to diabetes (first pregnancy with gestational diabetes), the nurse must remember to pick and choose what is taught and add to that body of knowledge later to avoid overwhelming the client. "Learning ability plateaus and time is needed to process information already learned before there is interest and motivation to learn more" (see Table 7.2). One last motivating point to use with pregnant women and young mothers is the fact that they can be positive role models in families living with diabetes.

Genetic Implications of Diabetes

In the beginning of this book, I discussed my guilt for bringing this disease into my family and adding to the list of familial diseases in my children's medical history. After some research, I discovered that their risk of contracting type 1 diabetes was very small.

Diabetes is caused by genetic factors and environmental factors. Most type 1 diabetics have inherited risk factors from both parents. It is also more prevalent in the White race. In order for this genetic factor to become manifest, there must be an environmental trigger. Research studies have isolated cold weather and certain viruses as possible triggers. Breast-feeding infants and feeding solids only after 6 months of age seems overprotective. Nurses should encourage all new mothers to breast-feed and delay solid foods, but this advice may have greater significance to women with type 1 diabetes. Breast-feeding also decreases insulin needs. Because this is an autoimmune disease, those who may get type 1 diabetes usually have autoantibodies in their blood. Siblings of type 1 diabetics could be tested for these autoantibodies to pancreatic beta cells.

Type 2 diabetes has a much stronger genetic component. A family history of type 2 diabetes is a very strong risk factor for getting the disease, however other components, such as obesity, a high-fat, low-fiber diet, and a sedentary lifestyle may make the difference between one family member who develops the disease and another who does not. Women who are diagnosed with gestational diabetes more often than not were infants of a mother with gestational diabetes (Dabelea et al., 2005).

The American Diabetes Association lists on their Web site (http://www. diabetes.org/genetics.jsp) the following genetic statistics. A child of a person with the listed characteristics has the following chance of developing the same type of·diabetes:

1. male with type 1 → child 1 in 17
2. female with type 1 birthing child before age 25 → child 1 in 25
3. female with type 1 birthing child after age 25 → child 1 in 100
4. both parents have type 1 diabetes → child between 1 in 10 and 1 in 4
5. male or female with type 2 diagnosed before age 50 → child 1 in 7
6. type 2 diagnosed after age 50 → child 1 in 13
7. both parents with type 2 → child 1 in 2

The prevalence of type 2 diabetes in some families is clearly genetic as well as learned behavior. Families often teach children by example including behavior such as poor food choices as well as avoidance of physical activity. Convincing a parent to turn this around for his or her children's sake, as well as controlling his or her own diabetes, could be very empowering for the client and the nurse.

DIABETES IN THE ELDERLY

The pancreas is an organ that ages along with the rest of the body. Its long-term function is related to how healthy it has always been and how old it is. I heard someone say once that 80% of 80-year-olds have type 2 diabetes as do 90% of 90-year-olds. If this is true, then the longer one lives, the more likely one is to have a pancreatic failure resulting in insufficient insulin to remain euglycemic. Some people in their 80s have had diabetes for decades and others have just been diagnosed. Most have type 2 diabetes but some have type 1, even if newly diagnosed. What this population knows and understands about diabetes self-management runs the gamut, from outdated information and even old wives' tales to completely correct information. Assessment of this population's knowledge base is as crucial to successful teaching as it is with any other age group. Additionally, the elderly may be experiencing comorbid conditions such as cardiovascular disease, arthritis, or visual and hearing impairment. Nurses need to adjust their teaching and expectations to accommodate any physical conditions an older person may be dealing with. Diabetes may or may not be his or her most important concern. Tight glycemic control should not be a goal if anyone already has end-stage renal disease or severe vision loss because the purpose of working at tight control is to prevent these and other long-term complications. Hypoglycemia can cause falls, strokes, and heart attacks in the elderly. When advocating for good glycemic control to prevent complications in 10 or 20 years, life expectancy is an issue. For someone to want to control a chronic disease in order to increase healthy longevity, life has to be worth living. If a small piece of pie or cake a few times a week puts a smile on an 80-year-old's face, he or she might be convinced to give up other carbohydrates at that same meal. Bargaining with older people is a teaching strategy worth exploring.

Overall, nutrition in the older population is often not assessed. Some elderly continue to eat well-balanced meals as long as someone provides them, such as in an elder care facility, through Meals on Wheels, or by living with a son or daughter. Eating is a social event. When taste buds and sense of smell decrease and energy level to cook wanes, the only pleasure in eating may be the company and conversation. The problem may not be an unwillingness to follow the diet but loneliness. Exercise is also more enjoyable in a group. Older people who participate in dancing, low-impact aerobics, and other group activities do so because it is fun, not because it helps to regulate blood sugar. All someone might need is encouragement to join a dance or aerobic group for their age level with the benefit of making new friends.

Good glycemic control, meaning an A1C of less than 7%, is recommended for most older people who don't have comorbid diseases. Testing blood sugars regularly is one means of achieving this goal. This should be taught using a meter commensurate with a person's physical and visual abilities. Many older persons have difficulty putting a strip in the tiny slot of the meter, so one that contains the strips and produces one at the touch of a button is helpful. Lancing devices should be easy to use and produce a small prick, making it less painful and preventing blood from going everywhere. Most older persons take aspirin daily to prevent clots, so finger sticking can get messy. It also helps to use a strip that requires a small amount of blood. Rationale for testing blood sugar needs to be convincing. One that I use means ruling in or ruling out hypo- or hyperglycemia when the patient does not feel well and helps them to determine what to do next. That is a good strategy for anyone with diabetes but is very motivating for seniors. Another is the fact that research demonstrates lowering blood glucose levels improves memory and the ability to concentrate, and increases one's enjoyment of life (Sakharova & Inzucchi, 2005). For some this might be very motivating. Just getting older people to consider their options and discuss their fears and concerns may improve the odds that they will follow through with what they have learned.

Some elders need more time to process information but may resent being talked down to. Demonstrating respect for their years of survival on this earth may be as simple as listening to how they used to have to boil glass syringes and sharpen needles, or how the first-generation oral agents made them feel, or how surviving diabetes without blindness or amputations years ago was considered a miracle. Anyone who has lived over half a century has stories to tell and wisdom to share. It takes longer to repeat instructions again and again than it does to listen to stories of the past in exchange for an attentive 10–20 minutes of learning about some aspect of diabetes self-management.

Medication is another area of concern for seniors with diabetes. A person does not have to have nephropathy to have decreased renal function. Aging causes loss of nephrons, so medication is not excreted as easily as it had been. Nurses need to access symptoms of medication accumulation. During and immediately after any illness, older persons should be watched for uncharacteristic changes in mood and behavior. Somnolence, lethargy, irritability, irrational thought, hallucinations, and confusion that is atypical if reported by family or friends need to be taken seriously because they may mean an accumulation of drug levels in the body. Recovery time from any ailment is usually prolonged, and an older person may need a referral to a home health agency for a while or may need supervision preparing and taking medication.

In doing research for this chapter, I was particularly interested in the recommendation for continuing use of insulin pumps with the elderly. Many older persons cannot achieve glycemic control without insulin. Herman and colleagues (2005) found that older type 2 diabetics with a mean disease duration of 16 years were able to achieve glycemic control of less than 7% from an average A1C of 8% or higher with either multiple insulin injections or use of an insulin pump.

Both groups experienced only a minimal number of mild (self-treated) hypoglycemic episodes and were satisfied with the treatment and the results. These clients had no cognitive impairments nor did they have any severe impairment of cardiac, liver, or rental function. This demonstrates what was stated in chapter 4 concerning the progressive nature of type 2 diabetes. In order to achieve A1C of less than 7%, most will eventually need insulin therapy. In this study group, both multiple injections of insulin and insulin delivered by pump did the job and provided client satisfaction.

All of the learning principles described in chapter 7 are applicable to both groups discussed in this chapter. How they are used with each group and with individuals within each group depends on a thorough assessment of each individual and the creativity of the nurse in applying the data collected to each one of the principles. The results are certainly worth the effort.

REFERENCES

American Diabetes Association. (n.d.). *Gestational diabetes.* Retrieved February 18, 2006, from http://www.diabetes.org/gestational-diabetes.jsp

American Diabetes Association. (2006). Standards of medical care in diabetes—2006. *Diabetes Care, 29,* S4–S42.

Barbour, L. A., & Friedman, J. E. (2003, March 6). Management of diabetes in pregnancy. *EndoText.com.* Retrieved March 11, 2006, from http://mdtext.com/diabetes/diabetes36/diabetes36.htm

Barss, V. A. & Repke, J. T. (2005, February 17). Patient information: Pregnancy complicated by pregestational diabetes. *UpToDate Patient Information.* Retrieved March 2, 2006 from http://www.patients.uptodate.com/topic.asp?file=pregnan/5061

Clausen, T. D., Mathiesen, E., Ekbom, P., Hellmuth, E., Mandrup-Poulsen, T., & Damm, P. (2005). Poor pregnancy outcome in women with type 2 diabetes. *Diabetes Care, 28,* 323–328.

Dabelea, D., Snell-Bergeon, J. K., Hartsfield, C. L., Bischoff, K. J., Hamman, R. F., & McDuffie, R. S. (2005). Increasing prevalence of gestational diabetes mellitus (GDM) over time and by birth cohort. *Diabetes Care, 28,* 579–584.

Herman, W. H., Ilag, L. L., Johnson, S. L., Martin, C. L., Sinding, J., Harthi, A. A., et al. (2005). A clinical trial of continuous subcutaneous insulin infusion versus multiple injections in older adults with type 2 diabetes. *Diabetes Care, 28,* 1568–1573.

Sakharova, O. V., & Inzucchi, S. E. (2005, November). Treatment of diabetes in the elderly. *Postgraduate Medicine, 118*(5). Retrieved March 11, 2006, from http://www.postgradmed.com/issues/2005/11_05/sakharova.htm

11

Diabetes and Mental Illness

Beverly Baliko

Mental illness is nothing to be ashamed of, but stigma and bias shame us all.

Bill Clinton

The National Institute of Mental Health (NIMH) estimates that over 26% of adult Americans experience a psychiatric disorder in any given year (Kessler, Chiu, Demler, Merikangas, & Walters, 2005). Of these, approximately 6% suffer from a serious and disabling mental illness, and nearly half meet diagnostic criteria for two or more disorders. According to the World Health Organization (2004), Major Depressive Disorder is the leading cause of disability in the United States for people ages 15–44.

With the prevalence of these psychiatric disorders, it is inevitable that some of the estimated 20.8 million Americans with diabetes (NDIC, 2006) will suffer from at least one mental illness at some point in their lives, potentially worsening these individuals' overall prognoses and increasing their health care costs. Compounding the problem, there is evidence that the emotional burden of diabetes, as well as its metabolic effects, may negatively impact mental health. There are also increasing concerns that certain medications commonly used in the treatment of psychiatric disorders can contribute to the development of diabetes or complicate disease management.

Severe mental illnesses such as major depression, bipolar disorder, and schizophrenia adversely affect individuals' cognition, functioning, communication, and motivation, sometimes making it more difficult for these clients to seek and receive adequate care, either for their psychological or physiological symptoms. The fragmentation and specialization within the health care system often create a barrier to comprehensive care. Other barriers can be internal, related to clients' knowledge and perceptions about their situations.

Sometimes when people recognize emotional problems and seek help, financial constraints can interfere with the ability to receive timely and appropriate care. In spite of all the popular rhetoric about the mind-body connection and the publicized information about the detrimental impact of stress on physiological functioning and the immune system, mental health treatment is undervalued for its adjunctive potential in the management of chronic health conditions. Most insurance plans have special caveats and limitations regarding mental disorders compared to other illnesses, with lifetime capitations, higher deductibles, and limited treatment options often the norm.

Though the concurrent management of mental disorders and diabetes clearly presents a challenge, the challenge can be met with knowledge, initiative, effective communication among providers, and careful health monitoring. A holistic approach that results in effective diagnosis and management of both psychological and physiological conditions can help prevent complications of each and improve the client's general well-being. In this chapter, we will examine the implications of two of the most problematic psychiatric symptoms—depression and psychosis—in terms of the management of diabetes and how nurses may best impact the care of individuals who suffer from comorbid physical and psychiatric conditions.

DIABETES AND DEPRESSION

The presence of any chronic or severe illness, including diabetes, may increase an individual's risk for development of a depressive disorder. Conversely, depression may have a negative impact on physiological disease outcomes by lowering immunity and interfering with individuals' ability and motivation to engage in healthy self-care practices and manage treatment regimens. Independent of the psychological effects of disease, there is growing evidence that the neuroendocrine changes involved in depression are themselves risk factors for the development of physiological illnesses such as cardiovascular disease and diabetes.

Research has indicated that people with diabetes are up to twice as likely as those without to suffer from depression (Anderson, Freedland, Clouse, & Lustman, 2001). Other studies have suggested that people who have both depression and diabetes are more likely to experience diabetes-related complications (deGroot et al., 2001). Depression is associated with poor glycemic control and problems with adherence to self-care regimens in terms of medications, exercise, smoking cessation, and diet (Lin et al., 2004; Lustman, Freedland, Griffith, & Clouse, 2000).

There is strong evidence that the risk is most increased in the presence of other physiological comorbidities in addition to diabetes and depression, an important finding because people with diabetes frequently have other chronic conditions (Egede, Nietert, & Zheng, 2005). Numerous studies have indicated that in patients with coronary artery disease (CAD), depression is associated with a 1.64 increased relative mortality risk (Joynt, Whellen, & O'Connor, 2003). This association has a biological etiology in the effect of depression on platelet characteristics, neuroendocrine activity, and heart function. Because 70–80% of people with diabetes die of CAD, this is another important finding. Haffner, Lehto, Ronnemaa, Pyorala, and Laakso (1998) found that the risk of myocardial infarction for individuals with diabetes with no prior diagnosis of CAD was the same as for nondiabetic people with a prior history of myocardial infarction.

The Chicken or the Egg?

The association between diabetes and depression is well established, but the nature of the relationship is not well understood. It was long assumed that depression, related to the ongoing situational stress of managing a chronic illness, followed diabetes. However, sometimes it may be the other way around or, at least, the relationship may be bidirectional. Altered glucocorticoid levels related to diabetes can affect brain function, but depression is also independently associated with elevated glucocorticoids in the brain, which might complicate diabetes. Depression, on the other hand, can lead to altered biochemical activities in the brain that are associated with insulin resistance (Barden, 2004).

Researchers who conducted a large study in Canada (Brown, Majumdar, Newman, & Johnson, 2005) discovered that, among 20- to 50-year-olds, people with newly diagnosed diabetes (type 2) were 30% more likely to have had a history of depression than people without diabetes, suggesting that the presence of depression may have increased the risk for these individuals. Interestingly, the difference did not hold true for older adults.

So, which comes first, the diabetes or the depression? The answer is that no one really knows, but it may be that several circumstances can contribute to individual risk. Among these are the stress resulting from disease management, discomfort associated with symptoms, the metabolic effects of the disease itself on the brain, factors such as age or the presence of other chronic illnesses, and even genetics. Genes have been identified that predispose individuals to both depression and obesity, the leading risk factor for type 2 diabetes. Regardless of the association, the nurse can play a critical role in interrupting the diabetes-depression cycle.

Challenges in the Management of Comorbid Depression and Diabetes

Depression presents significant health risks, especially for people who also have diabetes. The symptoms of depression often include fatigue, inactivity, appetite disturbance, forgetfulness, loss of concentration, and apathy, all of which can have serious consequences in the management of diabetes by negatively affecting treatment adherence and self-care practices. Not surprisingly, the focus on management of the physiological consequences of the disease process frequently overshadows concerns about the client's mental health. By the time a serious problem with depression is recognized, the client's overall health has suffered. Therefore, the recognition that depression is present is the first challenge in the management of diabetes and depression.

Diagnosis

Like it or not, the majority of individuals with problems such as depression and anxiety are going to present to their primary care provider, not a mental health professional. This could represent a reluctance by some people to admit to experiencing emotional problems or a lack of recognition of the problem as psychological in origin. Mental illness still carries with it a stigma. Clients, especially those who are older, of lower socioeconomic status, or of ethnic and racial minorities, are relatively unlikely to seek care for psychological issues until a situation becomes unbearable. Clients may even believe that emotional distress simply "comes with the territory" of coping with a chronic illness such as diabetes and may not bring up the topic unless the provider asks specific assessment questions. Although to some extent it is true that a degree of distress associated with coping with diabetes might be expected (information that is covered well in earlier chapters), when distress becomes persistent and interferes with functioning, more aggressive intervention may be necessary. Unfortunately, providers who share this assumption may tend to minimize or overlook signs of depression or anxiety.

What You Can Do

First, assess, assess, assess! Allow me a moment atop my soapbox: The lifetime prevalence of depression in the general population is so high (12-25%) that ALL patients should be routinely assessed for depression, but it is particularly important to include this type of assessment in the care of individuals with diabetes. Remember that you may be picking up on a condition that preexisted the diabetes or one that has been exacerbated or triggered by the presence of diabetes.

Many people with depression complain of fatigue, insomnia, or physical symptoms such as backache, headache, diarrhea, constipation, itching, or blurred vision. Such broad and overlapping symptoms can make accurate diagnosis more difficult, and providers may or may not be attuned to the potential for these types of symptoms to be warning signs of depression. Of course, a thorough assessment should include an evaluation of whether the depressive symptoms could be caused by medications or an interaction of medications that the client might be taking. This could be particularly important for clients with multiple conditions. Many medications, including antihypertensives, steroids, and hormones, can contribute to depression for some clients. One listing of such medications can be obtained online at http://www.medicinenet.com/script/main/art.asp?articlekey = 55169.

There are numerous brief tools that can be used to screen for depression (Valente & Saunders, 2005). These can be self-administered and may even be presented to patients with routine check-in paperwork. One easy tool—the Patient Health Questionnaire (PHQ-9)—was designed to be used in a primary care setting and can be accessed online at http://www.depression-primarycare.org/clinicians/toolkits/materials/forms/phq9/. In a recent encouraging reimbursement shift, one insurance company has piloted a program for primary care providers to screen high-risk clients for depression using the PHQ-9 (Moran, 2006). High-risk individuals are identified as those with with diabetes, coronary artery disease, or other chronic medical conditions. Even more simply, asking two questions assessing whether the client has experienced either of the two critical features of depression ("Over the past 2 weeks, have you felt down, depressed, or hopeless?" and "Over the past 2 weeks, have you felt little interest or pleasure in doing things?") can alert the provider to the need for further investigation and may be as accurate at detecting depression as lengthier tools (Whooley, Avins, Miranda, & Browner, 1997). These questions can easily be incorporated into the routine intake information. Should either of the answers be affirmative, it is critical that your assessment include questions concerning thoughts of death or suicide. Sometimes people respond to passive suicidal thoughts by neglecting their own care or taking health risks and to active suicidal thoughts by overdosing on potentially lethal medications. The risks of such a scenario involving a person with diabetes are apparent.

All clients should be asked about a personal and family history of depression. Depression has a high recurrence rate (60–90%), and there may be a genetic predisposition to the development of depression within families. This information can alert you to clients who may benefit from close monitoring.

Next, be sure that your clients with diabetes, and their families, recognize the signs of depression and the importance of seeking help promptly if depression is suspected. This type of education can be included in diabetes teaching and reinforced throughout the ongoing care process. Don't be afraid that bringing up the subject will somehow bring on a depression in a vulnerable or suggestible client. Instead, with this knowledge, you are providing the client with one more tool to optimize his or her own well-being. If you sense that your client is hesitant to admit to experiencing emotional problems, emphasizing the prevalence of depression and focusing on its biological origin can sometimes help increase his or her comfort level.

Nurses can work with other health care providers to ensure that clients receive appropriate treatment. Assessment for and detection of a problem is pointless unless it is addressed. Treatment should be individualized to the client's circumstances, symptoms, and preferences. Typical interventions include antidepressant medications, stress-management modalities, and psychotherapy. Often, individuals can be effectively treated for depression in the primary care setting, but a referral to a mental health professional may be warranted, especially in cases of severe depression or in the presence of suicidal thoughts. Diabetic clients can safely take antidepressants but should be followed carefully because of the potential side effects of the medications. Selective serotonin reuptake inhibitors (SSRIs) can increase risks of hypoglycemia, while tricyclic antidepressants (TCAs) are associated with hyperglycemia. Monoamine oxidase inhibitors (MAOIs), another class of antidepressants, can contribute to hypoglycemia and also require dietary restrictions that would be an additional burden to a client who is already coping with managing a diabetic diet. An adverse effect of antidepressant use that is particularly of concern for clients with diabetes is weight gain, but this is typically less of a problem for clients using SSRIs. Also, SSRIs may be a useful adjunct to the treatment of diabetes in that, in some cases, they produce an increase in insulin sensitivity (Goodnick, 2001; Lustman et al., 2000). Therefore, the diabetes medication regimen may require adjustment during antidepressant therapy.

Finally, it should also be noted that antidepressant therapy can decrease the symptoms of diabetic neuropathy for some clients (Goodnick, 2001; McDonald, 2004). Some of the same neurotransmitters responsible for regulating mood also have a role in the transmission of pain signals in the brain. It is important to emphasize to clients that these medications do not treat or inhibit the progression of neuropathy, so maintenance of their prescribed diabetes management regimen is imperative.

DIABETES AND CHRONIC, SEVERE MENTAL ILLNESSES

Certainly depression can be both chronic and severe, but mental illnesses that involve psychotic symptoms and more pronounced interference with cognition and thought processes can be even more challenging both for clients to cope with and for providers to treat. Fortunately, these disorders are less prevalent than depression. Approximately 1% of the world's population suffers from schizophrenia, and the estimates for the prevalence of bipolar disorder are around 3% (Kessler, Chiu, Demler, Merikangas, & Walters, 2005). Studies of comorbidities in people with chronic and severe mental illnesses indicate that about half suffer from known physical disorders and possibly another 35% have undiagnosed conditions (Felker, Yazel, & Short, 1996). These psychiatric disorders are not typically managed solely by the primary care provider because care often involves complex medication regimens and clients are less likely to be independent in following up with their own care. The care of such clients is traditionally fragmented. Attention to the more overt symptoms exhibited by clients with chronic mental illnesses means that physical symptoms do not take priority in the treatment plan, and lack of coordination of care often results in inadequate treatment for the physical health needs of these clients.

In terms of health care and community services, people with chronic mental illnesses are truly marginalized. The symptoms of their disorders often prevent them from following through with their own routine health care. Many live in adult group homes, or are homeless, with little psychosocial support. They receive their health care in clinics and agencies that accept Medicaid compensation or provide free services, which are generally limited in human and material resources. Deinstitutionalization and the closing of many long-term psychiatric beds has contributed to a large population of mentally ill individuals who are poor and whose multiple psychiatric and physical illnesses lead to deficits in functioning and self-care. So, access, financial constraints, and the disease processes are major barriers to adequate management of diabetes and other illnesses for those with chronic, severe mental illnesses.

Studies have shown that the chronic mentally ill population experiences higher rates of most diseases, but cerebrovascular, cardiovascular, endocrine, and pulmonary disorders are the major physiological contributors to the excess mortality rate (about double the general population) of individuals with chronic and severe mental illnesses (Kennedy, Salsberry, Nickel, Hunt, & Chipps, 2005). Prevalence rates for diabetes are reported as up to 14% in individuals with schizophrenia and up to 26% in those with bipolar disorder (Vreeland & Kim, 2004). When working and teaching in inpatient psychiatric settings, I have been struck by the number of clients with hypertension and diabetes, often not well controlled.

Numerous factors contribute to higher morbidity and mortality. As with depression, psychosis can contribute to an imbalance of corticosteroids, affecting glucose utilization in the body. One study suggested that increased visceral adiposity might be an inherent characteristic of schizophrenia, further affecting metabolism (Thakore, Mann, Vlahos, Martin, & Reznek, 2002). Detrimental lifestyle habits, such as poor diet, sedentary activities, and smoking, are associated with chronic and severe mental illnesses and are—as we know—risk factors for type 2 diabetes. The incidence of obesity is high, which is a problem in itself, and increases people's risk for other illnesses. A lack of health-promoting behaviors is one side of the coin, but unfortunately, medications used to treat psychiatric disorders are notorious for contributing to weight gain. This is particularly an issue for clients controlling their symptoms with mood stabilizers, such as lithium and the valproates (e.g., Depakote), and antipsychotic medications. The weight gain is a common reason that clients cite for lack of adherence to their prescribed psychotropic medication regimens (the most frequent cause of relapse). Weight loss programs are not routinely available in mental health settings. The medications also tend to cause dry mouth and increase thirst, leading to an excessive intake of sugar-laden beverages.

Antipsychotic Medications and Hyperglycemia

Of particular concern in recent years is the increasing evidence that several of the newer generation of antipsychotics contribute to the development of type 2 diabetes, not just by increasing the appetite and leading to weight gain, but through inducing metabolic changes and increasing insulin resistance. The diabetes may persist even with medication changes, probably because the antipsychotic medications are only one piece of the equation. These medications were welcomed and widely used because they seemed to have a lower risk of extrapyramidal side effects (movement disorders), were less sedating, and treated a wider range of symptoms than the older antipsychotic medications, such as haloperidol. There are only a few of these newer medications, and some are more likely to have adverse effects than others. According to the American Diabetes Association et al. (2004), an increased risk for the development of diabetes and dyslipidemia was associated with the use of clozapine (Clozaril) and olanzapine (Zyprexa). Discrepant results were found with the use of risperidone (Risperdal) and quetiapine (Seroquel), although these medications also contributed to weight gain. The newest medications, aripiprazole (Abilify) and ziprasidone (Geodon), had the least effect on weight and metabolic processes, but it is important to note that these do carry risks of other side effects, some potentially serious. Switching to the older antipsychotics is not an easy solution, because they, too, have long been associated with an increased rate of diabetes.

Does this mean that atypical antipsychotic medications should be avoided for clients with diabetes? Not necessarily. Current recommendations (and common sense!) are that baseline assessments of weight and metabolic status be obtained, especially for anyone with risk factors for diabetes or diagnosed diabetes, with regular monitoring during administration of the medications. Clients should also be monitored for symptoms of hypoglycemia, indicating a possible need to adjust their diabetes medications or inappropriate self-administration of medication. Symptoms such as confusion, fatigue, loss of concentration, and depressed mood can be misinterpreted as medication side effects or psychiatric symptoms. Clients certainly should not have to choose between controlling their diabetes or their psychotic symptoms, but the coexistence of both problems translates into a need for knowledgeable coordination of care to manage both conditions.

What You Can Do

Nurses can take an active role in monitoring lab work, noting symptoms that clients may exhibit and promoting early intervention. Perhaps in no population is your role as client advocate more critical. As a client advocate, you can communicate with other providers, document findings thoroughly, and do your best to ensure that clients' symptoms are adequately evaluated and that clients receive appropriate treatment. Unless you are an advanced practice psychiatric nurse, your involvement in direct intervention for the client's psychiatric illness may be minimal, but understanding this aspect of the client's care will better equip you to approach the client as a whole person rather than as a group of serious diagnoses. Updating yourself on psychiatric disorders you may have first heard about in nursing school and increasing your awareness of the potential implications of the use of psychotropic medications for clients with diabetes can give you a baseline upon which you can individualize care based upon each client's needs. A quick note: if you are going to be working with clients with severe and chronic mental illnesses, take stock of your own beliefs and opinions, fears and concerns about interacting with them, so that your own anxiety does not hinder your effectiveness.

TEACHING AND MOTIVATING CLIENTS
WITH MENTAL ILLNESSES

If your client is profoundly depressed, acutely psychotic, or severely anxious you will have to wait until these symptoms are controlled before any teaching interventions will be effective. Approach clients with patience and a nonjudgmental attitude. Really listen to them, acknowledge their feelings, whether or not you believe they are realistic, and let them know that their concerns have been heard. Avoid arguing, trying to convince them that they should feel differently, or minimizing their feelings—this invalidates them. Avoid false reassurances: "You'll feel a lot better once you learn how to work this glucometer." (The likelihood is that YOU are the one who will feel better.) These approaches will help clients to feel safe in honestly sharing their feelings.

Try to elicit their beliefs about mental illness and about diabetes. This allows you to approach the situation from their perspective and to offer information that can dispel misconceptions. Clients with mental illnesses often have low self-esteem, leading them to feel helpless and ineffectual. They may not feel competent to perform required self-care. You can help to counteract this tendency to focus on limitations by pointing out what they are doing well. Provide ongoing encouragement and let them know that you believe they can be capable collaborators in their own health care.

Loss of concentration, difficulty making decisions, and slowed thought processes are other common symptoms. Present your information in short spurts. Clients will not be able to take in a lot of complex information at once. Understand that more repetition and time than usual may be necessary to ensure that they comprehend the information. If they are not readily able to demonstrate their understanding to you, it does not mean they were being inattentive. Allow time for what you are saying to sink in and for questions to be formulated and asked. If you are working with a client who has a chronic and severe mental illness, you have to be prepared for ongoing teaching. Because of problems with cognition related to their illnesses and understanding of their medication regimens, such clients generally need frequent reinforcement of information.

Realize that low motivation, apathy, and low energy levels are prominent symptoms of many mental illnesses. If your client also has impairment in cognition and concentration, it is imperative to be sure that the client will have frequent follow-up and support in his or her self-care efforts. Successful control of symptoms is much more likely with the involvement of supportive family members or others.

You are already aware of the importance of teaching clients with diabetes about diet and exercise to help promote glycemic control. You can point out to clients that healthy diets and exercise also have the benefit of improving mood and decreasing fatigue. Strenuous exercise programs are not likely to be met with much success, but short intervals of exercise, walking, and noncompetitive activities can be helpful. It is important to remember that even minimal weight loss and exercise can have a beneficial effect. If you are able to help the client persist in healthier lifestyle behaviors long enough to exact a sense of improved well-being, the likelihood of maintaining the behaviors is improved. Engaging significant others in this effort or facilitating the involvement in interactive leisure activities in the community can help decrease isolation and encourage health-promoting habits.

Factors such as the amount of social and family support people receive, their previous coping skills, their beliefs about diabetes, and their own ability to manage their self-care can impact people's adjustment to a diagnosis of diabetes or the long-term management of diabetes. Conditions such as depression and anxiety can be short-lived or chronic. The potential stigma of mental illness should be acknowledged, and clients can be approached from the perspective of addressing overall well-being. Although many people are able to overcome debilitating psychological distress without professional intervention, we can do our best to ensure that they don't have to! Continued assessment is useful to minimize the impact of the distress and prevent the situation from worsening. Regular screening and prompt psychological interventions as needed should be incorporated into standard care. Nurses and other health care professionals can facilitate this by using brief standardized instruments, asking questions that elicit information about support, beliefs, and psychological distress associated with diabetes, and determining the degree to which distress impairs personal functioning. For individuals with known severe psychiatric disorders, it is critical to ensure that the disorders are adequately treated and resources for maximizing each individual's potential for self-care are in place.

REFERENCES

American Diabetes Association, American Psychiatric Association, American Association of Clinical Endocrinologists, North American Association for the Study of Obesity. (2004). Consensus development conference on antipsychotic drugs and obesity and diabetes. *Diabetes Care, 27,* 596–601.

Anderson, R. J., Freedland, K. E., Clouse, R. E., & Lustman, P. J. (2001). The prevalence of depression in adults with diabetes: A meta-analysis. *Diabetes Care, 24,* 1069–1078.

Barden, N. (2004). Implication of the hypothalamic-pituitary-adrenal axis in the physiopathology of depression. *Journal of Psychiatry and Neuroscience, 29*(3), 185–193.

Brown, L. C., Majumdar, S. R., Newman, S. C., & Johnson, J. A. (2005). History of depression increases risk of type 2 diabetes in younger adults. *Diabetes Care, 28,* 1063–1067.

deGroot, M., Anderson, R., Freedland, K. E., Clouse, R. E., & Lustman, P. J. (2001). Association of depression and diabetes complications: A meta-analysis. *Psychosomatic Medicine, 63*(4), 619–630.

Egede, L. E., Nietert, P. J., & Zheng, D. (2005). Depression and all-cause and coronary heart disease mortality among adults with and without diabetes. *Diabetes Care, 28,* 1339–1345.

Felker, B., Yazel, J., & Short, D. (1996). Mortality and medical comorbidity among psychiatric patients: A review. *Psychiatric Services, 47,* 1356-1363.

Goodnick, P. J. (2001). Use of antidepressants in treatment of comorbid diabetes mellitus and depression as well as in diabetic neuropathy. *Annals of Clinical Psychiatry, 13*(1), 31–41.

Haffner, S. M., Lehto, S., Ronnemaa, T., Pyorala, K., & Laakso, M. (1998). Mortality from coronary heart disease in subjects with type 2 diabetes and in nondiabetic subjects with and without prior myocardial infarction. *New England Journal of Medicine, 339,* 229–234.

Joynt, K. E., Whellan, D. J., & O'Connor, C. M. (2003). Depression and cardiovascular disease: Mechanisms of interaction. *Biological Psychiatry, 54,* 248–261.

Kennedy, C., Salsberry, P., Nickel, J., Hunt, C., & Chipps, E. (2005). The burden of disease in those with serious mental and physical illnesses. *Journal of the American Psychiatric Nurses Association, 11,* 45–51.

Kessler, R. C., Chiu, W. T., Demler, O., Merikangas, K. R., & Walters, E. E. (2005). Prevalence, severity, and comorbidity of twelve-month DSM-IV disorders in the National Comorbidity Survey Replication (NCS-R). *Archives of General Psychiatry, 62*(6), 617–627.

Lin, E. H., Katon, W., Von Korff, M., Rutter, C., Simon, G. E., Oliver, M., et al. (2004). Relationship of depression and diabetes self-care, medication adherence, and preventive care. *Diabetes Care, 27,* 2154-2160.

Lustman, P. J., Freedland, K. E., Griffith, L. S., & Clouse, R. E. (2000). Fluoxetine for depression in diabetes: A randomized double-blind placebo-controlled trial. *Diabetes Care, 23*(5), 618–623.

McDonald, K. (2004, October 25). Cymbalta—Treating depression and diabetic peripheral neuropathic pain. *Advance for Nurses,* p. 35.

Moran, M. (2006). Aetna to pay for depression screening by primary care physicians. *Psychiatric News, 41,* 5.

National Diabetes Information Clearinghouse. (2006). Total prevalence of diabetes in the United States, all ages, 2005. *National diabetes statistics.* Retrieved March 10, 2006, from http://www.diabetes.niddk.nih.gov/dm/pubs/statistics/index.htm

Thakore, J. H., Mann, J. N., Vlahos, I., Martin, A., & Reznek, R. (2002). Increased visceral fat distribution in drug-naïve and drug-free patients with schizophrenia. *International Journal of Obesity Related Metabolic Disorders, 26,* 137–141.

Valente, S. M., & Saunders, J. (2005). Screening for depression and suicide: Self-report instruments that work. *Journal of Psychosocial Nursing, 43,* 22–31.

Vreeland, B., & Kim, E. (2004). Managing the clinical consequences of psychiatric illness and antipsychotic treatmtent: A discussion of obesity, diabetes, and hyperprolactinemia. *Journal of the American Psychiatric Nurses Association, 10,* S17–S24.

Whooley, M. A., Avins, A. L., Miranda, J., & Browner, W. S. (1997). Case-finding instruments for depression: Two questions are as good as many. *Journal of General Internal Medicine, 12,* 439–445.

World Health Organization. (2004). *The World Health Report 2004: Changing history, Annex Table 3: Burden of disease in DALYs by cause, sex, and mortality stratum in WHO regions, estimates for 2002.* Geneva, Switzerland: Author.

12

Client Noncompliance

Nothing is a waste of time if you use the experience wisely.

Rodin

No book about teaching clients with chronic illness would be complete without a chapter on noncompliance. What is it and what can nurses do about it?

DEFINITIONS

Noncompliance means different things to different nurses. I was asked to speak to a group of nurses doing chronic disease management for a major insurance company as part of their in-service education. Out of a list of topics concerning diabetes, they chose "the noncompliant patient," as I thought they might. There is nothing more frustrating to a health care professional than to be rebuffed by a client after trying so hard to convince him or her to do what the nurse knows he or she ought to do to stay healthy. I had spoken to this group previously, and they knew that I had type 1 diabetes. Their list of definitions of what constituted non-compliance was very enlightening for me, as I fit many of them. They included the following:

- not following physicians' orders
- not following the diabetic diet
- not taking medications as ordered
- not losing weight
- not testing blood sugars as often as requested
- not exercising as prescribed

On the other hand, my definition of noncompliance is "a knowledgeable and conscious decision by a person to reject all help and a total refusal to try in any way to do anything that might be helpful in preserving his or her life and preventing complications, both acute and chronic. In other words, a decision by the client to cause his or her own eventual death." No one can be helped as long as he or she feels this way. All a nurse can do is let this person know that you are available to help if and when the person changes his or her mind.

Linda Carpinito (2002) in *Nursing Diagnosis: Application to Clinical Practice* gives a different opinion. The diagnosis of noncompliance describes the client who wants to follow the medical advice given but cannot because of physiologic or situational constraints such as lack of understanding, paralysis, or financial deficits. She specifically states that this diagnosis should not be used if the patient has made an informed decision not to comply (Carpinito, 2002).

Although, since 1993, the Joint Commission on Accreditation of Healthcare Organizations (JCAHO) requires all health care agencies to document that patients and families are taught what they need to know to participate in decision making concerning their health, there is little accountability on the patient to demonstrate behavior change based on this teaching (Rankin, Stallings, & London, 2005). Maybe that is what frustrates nurses so much. They do their part by teaching and yet some clients don't seem to want to participate in their own care. Some of the reasons why noncompliance occurs can be summed up under the two categories of "can't" and "won't."

FINANCIAL CONSIDERATIONS

Under the "can't" category there are many valid reasons why clients do not comply with instructions given. Diabetes is a very expensive disease. Blood glucose strips cost a dollar or more each, which may limit the number of times a client is able to test his or her blood sugar. Clients are also frustrated when they "waste" a strip if they get an error message instead of a glucose number and may be reluctant to use strips to do glucose controls on their meter. Human insulin costs $50 a vial, and the cost is more than $60 for newer human insulin analogs, such as Humalog, Novolog, and Lanthus. Even with a prescription drug card, co-pays can be substantial.

This may influence the number of injections and amount of insulin taken. The same applies to newer oral agents prescribed to control diabetes. It is embarrassing for some to admit they cannot afford to comply with medical orders or that they need help seeing or taking medications. This is especially true of older clients. Nurses can help them to troubleshoot these difficulties by asking open-ended questions about how they manage their health in a concerned and respectful manner. Many drug companies will provide medication with a physician's prescription to those who qualify for such assistance. Clients and/or family members can be directed to the Web site http://www.pparx.org for the Partnership for Prescription Assistance. (See chapter 4 for other helpful Web sites.) Many clients reuse syringes and lancets without adverse effects.

PHYSICAL LIMITATIONS

Clients may also not have the manual dexterity or visual acuity to use the meter they have or may not accurately draw up the correct dose of insulin, especially if two insulins are mixed, which often leads to uncontrolled blood sugars. Observing the client using his or her meter or drawing up insulin will provide the nurse with valuable insights as to what difficulties exist for this person in his or her self-care. The client and/or his or her family can be directed to the American Diabetes Association resource information guide at http://www. diabetes.org/diabetes-forecase/resource-guide.jsp for more appropriate meters that require less manual dexterity and have larger readouts. Pharmacies sell magnifiers that slide over syringes, and there are 30-unit syringes with more space between the lines, which increases the accuracy for small doses of insulin. If clients meet the Medicare criteria, a referral to home health agencies can be made by the physician. A home health nurse can prepare a week's supply of insulin in syringes that are then refrigerated and/or prepare a week's supply of medication in pill containers for this purpose. Pharmacies also provide these services and deliver the medication to the patient free of charge.

DEFICIENT KNOWLEDGE

The most common reason for lack of compliance under the "can't" category is lack of understanding. Too often, nurses make the assumption that a client with long-standing diabetes has learned what he or she needs to know. With short stays in hospitals, the initial instruction after the diagnosis of diabetes may have been overwhelming to the client and family and most of it may have been either not comprehended at that time or forgotten in the intervening years. Clients do not need nurses to repeat what was not understood the first time. Nurses should ask about how they deal with their diet, medication, and exercise to assess what is understood and what needs clarification and amplification.

LITERACY

Another reason for client ignorance concerning diabetes self-management is literacy. A client with a low literacy level can not comprehend most printed educational materials and may not understand the terminology used in educational videos. Assumptions are made that adults have a high school education, and teaching is done at that level using vocabulary and pamphlets that may not be appropriate. When clients fail to ask questions and avoid participation in discussions about their diabetes management, do not assume they are disinterested, have a flat affect, or consciously plan to disregard advice given. DeYoung (2003, p. 99) gives other behavioral examples of low literacy to watch for:

- not reading or even looking at printed material given
- stating that printed material will be shared with family members later
- claiming the need for eyeglasses that are broken or left at home
- stating they have a headache or are too tired to read over printed material
- mouthing words as they attempt to read anything written

My own mother, who dropped out of high school at the beginning of her junior year, hated to read and threw out printed instructions that did not have corresponding pictures. This did not diminish her intelligence but did significantly alter how she learned best. I was with her when she was admitted to the hospital once and watched as she convinced the nurse to fill out her medical history for her. After stating her birth date correctly, she then proceeded to add her age, 86, to that year to answer the question about today's date. The nurse misunderstood and said it was not 1986. I interrupted and told the nurse to wait until my mother finished her calculations. She got the year correct and knew it was close to Christmas. Not bad for someone who had been homebound for two years and never read the newspaper. It takes a great deal of assertiveness and self-esteem to interrupt a nurse or physician and ask that the discussion proceed in a simpler format. This is often too much to expect of older adults, immigrants with minimal English language skills, or those with less education. Even when asked if they understand what has been said, they verbalize understanding by nodding their head or saying, "yes." Why not request that they demonstrate understanding by asking them some what if questions? "What if you started to sweat and shake and were confused about what was happening to you? What would you do?" This encourages interaction, helps evaluate their vocabulary usage and problem-solving ability, as well as notes their understanding of the teaching on hypoglycemia. This must be done in a respectful manner so the client does not feel that the nurse is talking down to him or her. It is much more difficult to teach or interact with someone "not like us," including differences in age, education, culture, and experiences. It truly puts our ability to be understood by others to the test, a challenge we must accept if we are to reach others and have a meaningful impact on their lives.

CULTURE

Cultural differences can be huge obstacles to compliance with diabetes management. Culturally sensitive questions must be asked, using an interpreter if needed, to gather the data necessary to understand any barriers to compliance. "Cultural awareness is the process whereby the nurse becomes respectful, appreciative, and sensitive to the values, beliefs, and problem-solving strategies of a client's culture" (DeYoung, 2003, p. 79). We need to examine and recognize our own prejudices concerning other cultures and work at discarding them or, at least, blocking them from interfering with the care we give to others. Until nurses understand that they have those biases, they will not see how these biases interfere with the appropriateness of how they deal with members of another culture. By asking questions and gathering data through reading, workshops, or the Internet, nurses can begin to understand what cultural values and beliefs might interfere with client compliance. This openness to learning about a client's culture will help to break down barriers to meaningful communication. This open communication may need to start with the interpreter who may not translate everything that we say because he or she may be offended by or misinterpret instruction due to his or her own cultural bias. Speaking fluent English does not negate cultural upbringing. My father immigrated to the United States from Quebec, Canada, when he was 16, learned to speak English, and formed his own construction company. Despite this, his cultural beliefs concerning the need for preventative medicine and routine visits to doctors and dentists remained as it had been growing up on a farm in Canada. Doctors were called when someone was dying. By the time he saw a dentist for the first time in his 30s, he had no back teeth (all pulled out the old fashioned way with a string tied to a door knob). I have my wise though less educated mother to thank for insisting that my brother and I receive routine medical and dental care. When my father was diagnosed with lung cancer, resulting in a lobectomy and then radiation therapy, he asked no questions of the doctor. After talking to him, I discovered he had no understanding of how ill he was or how radiation could affect him. His oncologist told me that patients only ask when they are ready for the information. With my father's cultural background, he believed that the doctor would tell him what he needed to know. There was a large disconnect. On my insistence, his physician agreed to see my father again to explain in nonmedical terms what my father's situation was. However, he never asked him to repeat his understanding of it. On the way home, I did that using open-ended questions. That is the only way to evaluate another person's understanding, especially if he or she comes from a different cultural background.

In order to obtain culturally sensitive health care information from clients, DeYoung (2003) suggests variations of the following questions be incorporated in the interview:

- How do you explain the problem you have?
- What do you think caused this problem? (This is a question that should be asked of everyone.)
- When did it start?
- How does it make you feel?
- How bad is it?
- What are you afraid of most about this illness?
- What difficulties has it caused you at home, at work?
- How do you think it should be treated?
- What are the most important results you hope for from this treatment?

All of these questions may not be necessary in order to evaluate differences in cultural beliefs that could pose a communication problem between a health care practitioner and a client. One answer may lead to other more pertinent questions, but whatever is asked must be done in the spirit of acquiring the necessary information that will make teaching, learning, and disease management more likely.

RELIGIOUS CONSTRAINTS

If the client's religious beliefs prevent him or her from following through with prescriptive measures to control blood sugars, the client may not be compliant. Again, open-ended questions concerning how religious beliefs impact treatment of diabetes might yield useful information. A client may believe this diagnosis is a punishment from God for past sins. This may lead to a lack of compliance with the treatment regimen because the belief may be that he or she must suffer and that attempts to control the disease are defying God's will. Prevention of complications may be a totally unholy pursuit. In high school, I actually had a nun preach about sinful touching of breasts and looking at oneself naked in the mirror. I didn't know much about breast self-exams at the time, but I have often wondered about the rate of breast cancer in the members of that order at that time. Other religious beliefs might influence a client to pray more or give service to others rather than work at something as self-centered as diabetes self-management. Some religions are distrustful of modern medical practices and believe in the power of spiritual healers and their remedies. Women in some religions and cultures are second-class citizens and may not be deemed worthy of the time and expense that control of diabetes entails. They may need the express permission of a male relative (husband, father, brother, son) to access the health care options that will keep them well. Nurses need to ask good questions to obtain this information and understand the constraints that may prevent compliance. There may be subtle ways to work around these religious constraints and free the client to make better self-management choices. Just because a nurse does not agree with something that is not the norm, he or she must still deal with its reality in the client's life.

SUPPORT SYSTEM

Whether or not a client with any chronic disease can cope mentally or physically with the regimen to maintain glycemic control depends a great deal on his or her support network. Negative interactions with family members and friends can make or break the greatest resolve to do what is needed to live a fulfilling life despite diabetes. In " 'They care but don't understand': Family Support of African American Women with Type 2 Diabetes," the authors interviewed several women who perceived a lack of understanding of their needs by members of their social network (Carter-Edwards, Skelly, Cagle, & Appel, 2004).

I experienced this after my own diagnosis with diabetes. Family and friends may want to help but do not understand the disease or know what the client needs from them. Nurses can help explain the disease process and treatment options, but they need to empower clients to ask for what they specifically need from each of their support persons. Sometimes it may be to back off or to treat them as they had prior to the diagnosis. It may also include avoiding tempting foods or drink that the client needs to minimize. No one wants to be treated as fragile or different, but pretending one does not have special needs after being diagnosed with diabetes is not an option. Helping clients to verbalize what irritates them and planning how to dialogue with significant others is useful. Asking, "How would you like your family/friends to treat you?" is a start. Then, "What can you do to make that happen?" would be the next step. Trial and error is a reality, and the more options nurses can help the client realize, the closer he or she might come to getting the support he needs.

Now for my favorite category for noncompliance—the "won'ts." When a client refuses to follow prescribed advice and you have ruled out all of the areas covered under the "can't" category, the following issues should be explored. Some of these reactions to a diagnosis are part of the grief stages described by Dr. Elizabeth Kübler-Ross and discussed in the introduction to this book using personal examples. Some are based on a client's personality and life experiences.

DENIAL

Denial is an unconscious defense mechanism that protects us from a threat to self. In order to deal with the perceived loss of health that a diagnosis of diabetes brings, most people react with shock and denial. By refusing to accept this diagnosis, getting a second opinion, or remaining in a dazed state, the mind bides its time and allows for reality to sink in slowly. When we are ready to begin coping with this new entity, we can then listen to instructions and learn what we need to do. This is normal coping strategy and needs to be indulged by healthcare professionals, at least for a while. During this time clients and/or family members can be taught what is needed to improve the immediate health problem or threat to life. They can learn to test blood sugar, give insulin, or take oral medication. What they may not be able to grasp is that diabetes is a chronic illness and that lifestyle changes and medication are for life. Denial becomes pathological only when it persists beyond this initial stage and interferes with the process of acceptance so necessary in achieving good glycemic control. Health care providers may contribute to this by stating that type 2 diabetes is the "mild" form, nothing to worry about. Clients may comment that they have a touch of sugar or that they don't really need to worry about what they eat or about losing weight. Taking oral agents to control diabetes is like taking a vitamin pill. It is "no big deal." This attitude increases resistance to using insulin because "going on the needle" works against their denial. I have spoken to several clients with type 2 diabetes on oral hypoglycemic agents or experiencing neuropathy and cardiovascular complication indicating years of hyperglycemia who state they have never been diagnosed with diabetes. Denial is very powerful and difficult to break through. Nurses can talk about good health care practices for everyone and focus on improving whatever clients are willing to deal with, like the numbness and tingling of feet or the decrease in circulation. Blood sugar control will improve or at least prevent further deterioration of their current condition. Giving them handouts concerning diet, exercise, medications, and weight loss that mention diabetes may be a nudge in the right direction. Listening to their thoughts about diabetes may uncover personal fears that they will become like a neighbor or relative who suffered and died of diabetic complications. Knowing what is behind this prolonged and unhelpful denial may give the nurse insight and information with which to formulate an offer the client can't refuse. If a client wants to do something specific with his or her life, like a career, family, sports, or longevity, he or she may fear that acceptance of this diagnosis will make it impossible. Now you have a tool to motivate the client to work at control in order to improve the odds that his or her dreams will be realized. Most people need to work at one thing at a time. Help the client choose which area he or she is willing to deal with first. It may be quitting smoking (diabetes and smoking is a deadly combination). This might lead to brisk walking because he or she has more energy and lung capacity, which usually results in weight loss.

ANGER

Anger is ever-present in most people diagnosed with a chronic illness. "Why me?" is always under the surface and can spring up even after years of good control. A client may state or act as if he or she just does not want to deal with "it" anymore or needs a break from doing blood sugars, counting carbs, and/or taking medication or insulin. Because type 1 diabetics will get very ill quickly if they stop taking insulin, their choice may be to eat whatever they want and stop testing their blood sugar for a few days or longer. It will quickly become apparent that this plan is making them sick and less able to enjoy life. Nurses can use this realization to reinforce the importance of glycemic control while understanding the client's need to take a vacation from the tedious regimen. People with type 2 diabetes can last much longer avoiding control before feeling bad. However, clients usually can talk about life changes that have happened over this noncompliant time, which they may relate to the aging process; changes discussed include decreased energy level, disinterest or lack of enjoyment in things that once held their attention, like sports or grandchildren, and falling asleep after eating. Once you know what they miss doing, you can use this to motivate them to return to good control. Some people use anger at diabetes to lash out at others, which causes problems with family and work relationships. Focusing on the cause of anger can help to vent feelings of frustration at having diabetes and being forced to change lifestyle. When I experience anger at diabetes, I always remember what a wise physician once said in the early days of my diabetic career: "Diabetics have to do what everyone else ought to do." Now instead of being angry, I feel challenged to lead a healthy lifestyle, to be an example to my family and peers, and to be a leader. How empowering!

Nurses need to be good listeners and encourage clients to get their feelings out. Once the issues bothering someone are on the table, the client can recognize them for what they are and begin to deal with them. As long as they remain inside, these issues simply cause agitation, anger, and frustration. To get a discussion going, ask, "What is it like to live with diabetes?" or "How does having diabetes make you feel?" If the client is experiencing anger, be prepared for him or her to let you really know in no uncertain terms. You may have opened up the floodgates bottled up for years. Always remember that the client's anger is not directed at you but at the disease. Once the flood of words has subsided, you can ask, "So what would you like to do about it?" You may have given him or her the first opportunity to come to grips with this new life change no matter how long it has been since diagnosis. Please remember that a client's anger can be a powerful force leading to new learning and growth in self-care. Listening and allowing the client to dump all of his or her pent-up emotions can be the catalyst for this change.

DEPRESSION

In the process of accepting the loss of good health, the loss of being "normal," whatever that means to an individual, or the diagnosis of a chronic illness, some sadness or depression is necessary. Without it people remain in the stages of denial and anger. As the reality of how life has been altered forever by a diagnosis of diabetes sets in, a client may withdraw from loved ones or display signs of hopelessness and helplessness even while doing some of the activities necessitated by the diagnosis. The client may check his or her blood sugar and give insulin or take oral medication but be unable to problem solve when blood sugars are not what they should be. Lack of energy may make physical activity impossible. Destructive behaviors like imbibing alcoholic beverages, smoking, or relying on mind-altering drugs (prescribed, over the counter, or illegal), may take over. Thoughts of suicide, the ultimate escape, may take center stage. Nurses need to evaluate whether the sadness and depressed mood exhibited by the client is part of the coming to terms that is a normal and expected phase of acceptance or a true situational depression necessitating psychiatric intervention. When in doubt, get an order for a psychiatric evaluation. Depression is covered in more depth in chapter 11.

FATALISM

"Traditional educational interventions are designed to give the same information to everyone and to teach new coping skills without first addressing the well-established beliefs that drive the selection of coping strategies" (Redman, 2004, p. 24). If there is a family history of diabetes with negative consequences, this diagnosis can either help a client do what relatives did not do or lead the client to believe that there is nothing he or she can do that will make his or her fate any different than that of others with diabetes complications. I have heard a variation of both themes from people diagnosed with diabetes. If a person concludes that his or her grandmother died of diabetic complication because she did nothing to control blood sugar, I know that person is open to learning how to prevent the same consequences from happening to him or her. If, however, they believe in the inevitability of similar consequences happening to them, I know I have my work cut out for me. People in the latter category have no incentive to make lifestyle changes or follow their blood sugars because they believe it will not make any difference in the long run. About 10 years ago, a family practice physician told me informally that he would rather die than take insulin injections. I answered that I felt sorry for his patients. According to the literature, this attitude is not uncommon and leads to more preventable long-term complications when type 2 diabetics are not switched to insulin if glycemic control is not achieved (Peyrot et al., 2005). This attitude on the physician's part may contribute to the fatalism that some with type 2 diabetes feel.

SELF-DETERMINATION

Many people with chronic illnesses develop strategies of self-management that differ from the prescribed regimens. They may use alternative therapies or alter when they take medications or do blood sugars. Some self-management strategies are stricter or more difficult than what is prescribed. All of these patients may be labeled noncompliant by their health care practitioner. In diabetes as in all other experiences in life, one size never fits all. Clients who want to manage their diabetes "my way" need to be in a collaborative relationship with health care providers. No one knows a person's history, beliefs, likes, and dislikes, and how his or her body deals with glycemic control better than the client. What clients need from nurses are tools to make good choices and cope with life and the ups and downs of blood sugars. When anyone asks me how often I check blood sugars, my answer is "as often as I need the information." That might mean 3 times a day or up to 10 times. I might need the information in the middle of the night or before I go for a walk. Clients need to be encouraged to test after meals, not just before meals. The real proof of control is whether a 2-hour postprandial blood sugar stays under 140 mg/dl.

There is so much written about diabetes today that health care practitioners need to realize they are not the only voice a client hears. Nurses need to know what their clients are reading and who they are listening to. Some of the recent offers I have received in the mail include titles from the American Diabetes Association, the Mayo Clinic, *Johns Hopkins White Papers,* and publication from *Diabetes Self-Management* as well as some of dubious value touting weight loss without dieting and exercise or the sugar cure for diabetes. The Web is also a source of well-researched and useful information, as well as personal opinions, product pushing "cures," and other unsubstantiated guides. We need to help clients evaluate these resources by asking them to note the author or organization contributing the information and the date when it was posted. Outdated information is not useful. Other questions to ask include the following: "Is the article selling something?" "Does it include studies proving the points made?" "And does it make sense?" If an article states what a client wants to hear, it may be too good to be true.

The proof of any self-management strategy is in the hemoglobin A_{1c}. There are clients that are compliant and have A1Cs above 7%. That may mean they are "cheating" or, more likely, the current medication regimen is inadequate. There are also clients who are considered noncompliant with A1Cs consistently below 7%. Nurses should conclude that these clients must be doing something right. In a recent article on patient compliance in *Family Practice Management,* the author states, "The physician has to recognize the opportunity for intervention, reframe it in a way that makes it meaningful to the patient and generate a sufficient sense of urgency to compel the patient to take action. At the same time, the physician has to maintain a partnership with the patient, based on trust and understanding" (Pawar, 2005, p. 44). I could easily substitute "the nurse" for the physician in this quote. In other words, nurses need to encourage discourse, listen carefully, use what the client says, and "make him an offer he cannot refuse." In order to convince the client to change, the nurse must "sell" good glycemic control in a way that the client can understand and that makes sense to him or her. The five tips given by Pawar (2005) to improve patient satisfaction and compliance include the following:

1. Establishing a trusting and caring relationship. Clients must believe we value them as people not just as work related charges.

2. Uncover patients' actual needs and concerns. Ask follow-up questions to get at the real issues that trouble the client.
3. Use dialogue, not monologue. Encourage participation and really listen to what clients say.
4. Don't force or threaten; little steps are better than nothing. Keep the client in charge of his or her own care. Ask "Are you willing to do blood sugars before each meal for 1 week?" Incremental steps are often needed.
5. Follow-up is paramount. This may be by phone if you see the client in an office or outpatient setting or it may be as simple as checking in on an inpatient client each day you are working, even if he or she is not part of your assignment.

If nurses were to use the above selling strategies and respect the right of clients to refuse or modify diabetes management strategies, they would look at their jobs with a greater sense of fulfillment and would experience less burnout. Hopefully, we, as nurses and health care professionals, will stop the ineffectual labeling of patients as noncompliant and realize that there is a reason, maybe even several, why a client cannot or will not comply with the medical regimen prescribed. Until we know and understand what these reasons are, we cannot help the client in his or her struggle to improve his or her diabetes self-management. Each time we work with a client who might be considered noncompliant, we cannot write him or her off. Trying some of the strategies listed in this book and any others that we can think of will help us learn from these challenges and work at perfecting our approach to such clients. We as nurses may never see the results of our efforts, but we know that we have given the client something to think about when no one else may have tried.

REFERENCES

Carpinito, L. J. (2002). *Nursing diagnosis: Application to clinical practice* (9th ed.). Philadelphia: Lippincott.

Carter-Edwards, L., Skelly, A. H., Cagle, C. S., & Appel, N. J. (2004, May-June). "They care but don't understand": Family support of African American women with type 2 diabetes. *Diabetes Education, 30*(3), 493–501.

DeYoung, S. (2003). *Teaching strategies for nurse educators.* Upper Saddle River, NJ: Prentice Hall.

Lippincott Williams Wilkins (2005). *Patient education in health and illness* (5th ed.). Philadelphia: Lippincott Williams and Wilkins.

Pawar, M. (2005). Five tips for generating patient satisfaction and compliance. *Family Practice Management, 12*(6), 44–46.

Peyrot, M., Rubin, R. R., Lauritzen, T., Skovlund, S. E., Snoek, F. J., Matthews, D. R., et al. (2005). Resistance to insulin therapy among patients and providers. *Diabetes Care, 28,* 2673–2679.

Redman, B. K. (2004). *Advances in patient education.* New York: Springer Publishing.`

Index

Page numbers in italic indicate tables.

Abilify. *See* Aripiprazole
Acarbose (Precose, Glucobay, Prandase), *30,* 34
Acceptance, by diabetes client, 151
Ace inhibitors, 122
Actos. *See* Pioglitazone
ADA. *See* American Diabetes Association
Adherence, 111, 131
Adolescents, with diabetes, 9, 107–112
Adult onset diabetes, 1
Adults with special needs, diabetes in, 115–127
Advocating, for diabetes client, 85, 138
Agency care, client education for, 83–85
Alcohol, 17–18, 58
Aldomet. *See* Methyldopa
Alpha cells, 4
Alpha-glucosidase inhibitors, *30,* 31–32, 34
Amaryl, *29,* 31, 33
American Diabetes Association (ADA), 12, 59, 79, 81, 94–95, 102, 106, 124, 145
   diabetes classification by, 1, 3
   recommendations by, 8–9, 13–14, 36, 51–53, 119–120

Amylin hormone, 44
Anger, of clients with diabetes, 152–153
Angiotensin receptor blockers (ARBs), 122
Antidepressants, 134–135
Antidiabetic medication. *See* Medication
Antipsychotic medications, 136–138
Anxiety. *See* Depression
Apidra. *See* Insulin glulisine
Approval, of new drugs or products, 71–74, *73,* 126, 133
Apresoline. *See* Hydralazine
ARBs. *See* Angiotensin receptor blockers
Aripiprazole (Abilify), 137
Assessment, of client, 82, 133–134, 140
Assistance, with drug costs, 27–28, 93, 145
AT-1001. *See* Zonulin inhibitor
Autoimmune destruction, prevention of, 65–67
Autonomy, of diabetes client, 82–84, 107–112
Avandadryl. *See* Avandia/glimeperide
Avandamet. *See* Rosiglitazone/metformin

Avandia. *See* Rosiglitazone
Avandia/glimeperide (Avandadryl),
33–34

Babies, with diabetes, 99–100
Basal insulin, 35
Beta-blockers, 58
Beta cells, 3–4, 6, 28, 66, 69–70
Biguanides, *30,* 31–32
Bipolar disorder, 129, 135–137
Birth defects, 116–117, 117
Blood glucose meters, 59, 145. *See
also* Continuous blood glucose
monitors
Blood sugar, 31–32, 108, 119, 121,
125–126
changes in, 3–5, 18
control of, 51–63
during exercise, 22–24
factors affecting levels of, 12–13,
54–58, *55*
hemoglobin A$_{1c}$ correlation with, *52*
high levels of, 53–56, 100, *101,*
104–105
low levels of, 56–59, 99–100, *101*
monitoring of, 59–63, 121,
125–126
testing of, 18–19, 119–120
See also Fasting blood sugar
BMI. *See* Body mass index
Body mass index (BMI), *15*
Bolus doses, 35, 40
Breast feeding, diabetes during, 123
Bumex, 56
Byetta. *See* Exenatide

CAD. *See* Coronary artery disease
Caffeine, 56
Caloric intake, 14
Camping, for adolescents with
diabetes, 111
Cancer, of pancreas, *5*
Carbohydrates, 34
counting of, 16–17

insulin matching with, 13, 16–17,
35–36
intake of, 12–13, 56–57, 121–122
Cardiovascular disease (CVD), 7–8,
12, 18, *25*
CD1d gene, 67
Cheating, 80, 104–105, 155
Children, with diabetes, 9, 97–106,
101
Chlorpropamide (Diabinese), 28
Cholestyramine (Questran), 33
Classification, of diabetes types, 1, 3,
5, 5–8
Client
autonomy of, 82–84, 107–112
concerns of, 83–85, 121–122, 156
lack of understanding by, 145–150
noncompliance of, 36, 80,
109–112, 143–156
patient v., 82–83
Client education, 79–95, 111, 134,
145–146
for diabetic clients with mental
illness, 138–140
for elderly with diabetes, 124–127
essential components of, 80–81, *81*
evaluation of, 93–95
goals of, 82–85
learning principles for, 85–93, *89,*
122–123
for pregnant clients, 120–123
Clinical trials, for new diabetes medication, 72–74
Clozapine (Clozaril), 137
Clozaril. *See* Clozapine
Coma, 54, 58
Combination agents, *30,* 32
Communication
with diabetic clients, 145–150
with toddlers with diabetes, 99–100
Comorbid conditions, with diabetes,
124–125, 129–140
Compliance, with diabetes management, 36, 80, 109–112, 143–156

Continuous blood glucose monitors,
61–63
Contracts, for adolescents with
diabetes, 110
Coping skills, 108, 111, 132–133,
150–154
Coronary artery disease (CAD), 131
Corticosteroids, 7, 56, 67, 136
Costs, of diabetes management,
27–28, 93, 144–145
Counting, of carbs, 16–17
Culture, client noncompliance
resulting from, 147–148
Cure, for diabetes, 65–74
CVD. *See* Cardiovascular disease
Cyclosporine, 80

Daclizumab, 68
Decision making, for diabetes
management, 83, 139
Denial, of clients with diabetes,
150–151
Depakote. *See* Valproates
Depression, diabetes and, 108, 110,
130–135, 153
Destructive behaviors, of clients with
diabetes, 153
DexCom STS Continuous Monitoring
System, 62
DiaBeta, *29,* 31
Diabetes
adolescents with, 107–112
in adults with special needs, 115–127
basics of, 3–9
children with, 9, 97–106, *101*
classification of, 1, 3, *5,* 5–8
client noncompliance in
management of, 36, 80,
109–112, 143–156
cure for, 65–74
depression and, 108, 110,
130–135, 153
diagnosis of, 3, 8–9, 52–53,
120, *120*

educating client on, 79–95
in elderly, 124–127
essential components for
management of, 80–81, *81*
genetics of, 123–124
glycemic control in, 35, 47, 51–63,
60, 108, 110, 116, 121,
125–127, 131, 154–155
learning principles for, 85–93, *89,*
122–123
medical nutritional therapy for,
11–19
medication for, 27–49
mental illness and, 129–140
physical activity for treatment of,
21–26
pregestational, 115–117
during pregnancy, *5, 7,* 36, 42, 56,
115–124
risk factors for, 6–9, *15,* 119–120,
131–132, 137
self-management of, 77–156
symptoms of, 8, 53, 97, 99
See also Gestational diabetes
Diabetes Education and Camping
Association, 111
Diabetes Forecast (ADA), 94–95
Diabetes Medical Management Plan
(DMMP), 100–102, *103*
Diabetes mellitus, 3
Diabetes mellitus client questionnaire,
90–91
Diabetes questionnaire, *86–88*
Diabinese. *See* Chlorpropamide
Diagnosis
of depression, 132–133
of diabetes, 3, 8–9, 52–53,
120, *120*
of metabolic syndrome, 71
Diet, 11–12
2005 Dietary Guidelines for
Americans, 15–16
Disability, from mental
illness, 129

Discrimination, against people with
diabetes, 102
Discussion, with diabetes client,
92–93, 146–147, 156
DMMP. *See* Diabetes Medical
Management Plan
Dosing
of glucagon, 59
of pramlintide, 44–45, *45*
D-phenylalanine derivatives, *29,* 31
Drinking, pros and cons of, 17–18
Drugs. *See* Medication

Eating disorders, in adolescents with
diabetes, 110
Edmondton Protocol, for
transplantation, 67–68
Education
of school children with diabetes,
100–104
See also Client education
Elderly, diabetes in, 124–127
Emotional problems. *See* Mental
illness
Environmental factors, of diabetes, 123
Environment, for learning, 92
Estrogen, 56
Evaluation, of teacher, 93–95
Exenatide (Byetta), 45, 46
Exercise, with diabetes, 21–26, *25*
Exubera. *See* Inhaled insulin

Family history, in diabetes, 123
Family, of clients with diabetes,
149–150
Fasting blood sugar, 116
ADA guidelines for, 52–53
for diabetes classifications, 3, *5,* 8
Fatalism, of clients with diabetes,
153–154
Fats, dietary, 12–14, 17
FDA. *See* Food and Drug
Administration
Feet, inspection of, 26

Fiber, 13, 17
Financial impact
of diabetes care, 93, 144–145
of mental illness, 130
504 Plan, 102
FlexPen. *See* Insulin mixtures
Follow-up, for diabetes client, 156
Food and Drug Administration
(FDA), drug approval by, *73,*
73–74
Food pyramid, 15–16
Friends, of clients with diabetes,
149–150

GDM. *See* Gestational diabetes mel-
litus
Genetics, in disease, 123–124, 132,
134
Geodon. *See* Ziprasidone
Gestational diabetes, *5,* 118–120, *120*
Gestational diabetes mellitus (GDM),
7, 119
Glimeperide (Amaryl), *29,* 33
Glipizide, *29*
Glipizide/metformin (Metaglip), *30,*
32
Glitazones. *See* Thiazolidinediones
Glucagon, 4, 46, 58
Glucobay. *See* Acarbose
Glucocorticoids, 131
Glucola, 7, 119
Glucophage, *30,* 33
Glucophage XR, *30,* 33
Glucose, 3–5. *See also* Impaired
fasting glucose; Impaired glucose
tolerance; Random blood glucose
Glucose challenge test, 7, 119
Glucose tablets, 24
Glucosuria, 53
Glucotrol, *29,* 31
Glucotrol XL, *29,* 31
Glucovance. *See* Glyburide/metfor-
min
GlucoWatch G2 Biographer, 63

Glumetza. *See* Metformin
Glyburide, *29*, 117, 122
Glyburide/metformin (Glucovance), *30*, 32–33
Glycemic control, 35, 47, 51–63, *60*, 108, 110, 116, 121, 125–127, 131, 154–155
Glycogen, 4, 31–32
Glycosylation, of hemoglobin, 51–52
Glynase PresTab, *29*, 31
Glyset. *See* Miglitol
Grief stages, 150
Guardian RT Continuous Glucose Monitoring System, 62

Haloperidol, 137
HCTZ. *See* Hydrochlorothiazide
Hemoglobin A1c, 47–49, 51–52, *52*, 62, 120–121, 155
Hexyl-insulin monoconjugate 2 (HIM2), 70
HIM2. *See* Hexyl-insulin monoconjugate 2
History. *See* Family history
Home health nurse, 145
Hormones, 56, 133
Hospitalization, diabetes and, 56, 83–85
Humalin L. *See* Lente insulin
Humalin U. *See* Ultralente insulin
Humalog. *See* Insulin lispro
Humalog Mix 75/25. *See* Insulin mixtures
Human incretin hormone GLP-1, 45–46
Human insulin, 37, 144
Humulin 50/50. *See* Insulin mixtures
Humulin 70/30. *See* Insulin mixtures
Humulin N. *See* NPH insulin
Humulin R. *See* Insulin
Hydralazine (Apresoline), 122
Hydration, during exercise, 25
Hydrochlorothiazide (HCTZ), 56
Hydrogenated oils, 13–14

Hyperglycemia, 3, 7, 35–36, 53–56, *101*, 116–117, 120, 135, 137–138
Hyperosmolar nonketosis, 54
Hypoglycemia, 18–19, 23–24, 28–35, 44, 48, 55–59, *101*, 122, 135, 137–138

IEP. *See* Individualized Education Plan
IFG. *See* Impaired fasting glucose
IGT. *See* Impaired glucose tolerance
Immunologic suppression, with transplantation, 67–68
Impaired fasting glucose (IFG), 7–9, 12, 52–53
Impaired glucose tolerance (IGT), 7–9, 12
IN-105, 70
Incretin mimetics, 45
Individualized Education Plan (IEP), 102–104
Inhaled insulin (Exubera), *38*, 46–49
Injections, for diabetes treatment, 34–46
Insulin (Humulin R, Novolin R, Novolin R PenFill), 32–35, 43, 46–49, *103*, 104, 123, 144–145
body's production and use of, 3–5, 28–31
carbohydrate matching with, 13, 16–17, 35–36
for diabetes treatment, 34–44
for elderly, 126–127
exercise with, 23–24
oral, 70
during pregnancy, 116, 122
types of, 37–40, *38–39*
Insulin analogs, 37, 40–41, 144
Insulin aspart (NovoLog, NovoLog Flexpen), *38*, 40
Insulin detemir (Levemir, Levemir Flexpen), *39*, 41
Insulin glargine (Lantus), *39*, 41
Insulin glulisine (Apidra), *38*, 40

Insulin lispro (Humalog), *38,* 40, 41
Insulin mixtures (Humulin 50/50,
    Humulin 70/30, Novolin 70/30,
    Novolin 70/30 PenFill, Novolin
    70/30 InnoLet, NovoLog 70/30,
    FlexPen, Humalog Mix 75/25), *39,*
    40–41
Insulin pumps, 35, 40, 42–44, 84–85,
    126–127
Insulin resistance, 6–7, 14, 32, 56, 71,
    108, 116, 119, 120, 131, 137
Intermediate-acting insulin, *38,* 58, *60*
Internet, for educating clients with
    diabetes, 111
Islet cells, 34–35, 65–69
Islets of Langerhans, 4

JDRF. *See* Juvenile Diabetes Re-
    search Foundation
Journaling for weight loss, 14–15
Juvenile Diabetes Research
    Foundation (JDRF), 66, 81
Juvenile onset diabetes, 1

Ketoacidosis, 6, 9, 43, 53–54, 116
Ketonemia, 36
Ketonuria, 23, 36, 53
Kidney, transplantation of, 67
Knowledge, for diabetes
    management, 88–89, 145–146
Kübler-Ross, Elizabeth, 150

Lactic acidosis, 32
Lantus. *See* Insulin glargine
Lasix, 56
Learning environment, 92
Learning principles, for nursing
    interventions, 85–93, *89,* 122–123
Lente insulin (Humulin L, Novolin
    L), 37, *38*
Levemir. *See* Insulin detemir
Levemir Flexpen. *See* Insulin detemir
Lifestyle, 12, 22–23, 61, 136,
    139–140

Literacy, client lack of, 146–147
Lithium, 137
Liver disease, 36
Liver function tests, with
    thiazolidinedione treatment, 32–33
Long-acting insulin, *39*

Major Depressive Disorder, 129
Management
    of comorbid depression and
        diabetes, 132
    in DMMPs, *103*
    of sick days, 18–19
    See also Self-management
Management plans, for school-age
    children with diabetes, 100–104
MAOIs. *See* Monoamine oxidase
    inhibitors
Meal planning, in DMMPs, *103*
Medical nutritional therapy, 11–19
Medication, 27–49, 56, 117–118
    approval of, 71–74, *73,* 126, 133
    costs of, 27–28, 93, 144–145
    for mental illness, 136–138
    new, 65–74
    during pregnancy, 122
Medscape, 49
Medtronic-MiniMed, 61–62
Meglitinides, 28–31, *29,* 32
Mental illness, diabetes and,
    129–140
Metabolic syndrome, 7–8, 71
Metaglip, *30,* 33
Meters. *See* Blood glucose meters
Metformin (Glucophage, Glumetza,
    Riomet), *30,* 31–34, 45, 118
Methyldopa (Aldomet), 122
Micronase, *29,* 31
Miglitol (Glyset), *30,* 34
Monitoring, of blood glucose, 59–63,
    121, 125–126
Monoamine oxidase inhibitors
    (MAOIs), 58, 135
Mood stabilizers, 137

Motivation, of diabetic clients,
120–123, 138–140
My pyramid, 15–16

Nateglinide (Starlix), *29,* 31, 57
National Diabetes Information
Clearing House (NDIC), 27
National Institute of Diabetes and
Digestive and Kidney Diseases
(NIDDK), 74
Natural killer (NKT) T cells,
66–67
NDIC. *See* National Diabetes
Information Clearing House
Nephropathy, *25*
Neuropathy, *25,* 135
Nicotinamide, 69
Nicotine, 58
NIDDK. *See* National Institute of
Diabetes and Digestive and Kidney
Diseases
Nifedipine (Procardia), 122
NKT T cells. *See* Natural killer T
cells
Noncompliance, with diabetes
management, 36, 80, 109–112,
143–156
Novolin 70/30. *See* Insulin mixtures
Novolin 70/30 InnoLet. *See* Insulin
mixtures
Novolin 70/30 PenFill. *See* Insulin
mixtures
Novolin L. *See* Lente insulin
Novolin N PenFill. *See* NPH insulin
Novolin R. *See* Insulin
Novolin R PenFill. *See* Insulin
NovoLog. *See* Insulin aspart
NovoLog 70/30. *See* Insulin
mixtures
NovoLog Flexpen. *See* Insulin aspart
NPH insulin (Humulin N, Novolin
N, Novolin N PenFill), 37, *38,* 40,
47, 80
Nurse, as teacher, 79–95

Nutrition, for diabetes treatment,
11–19, 121–122, 125

Obesity, 6, 14, 32, 120, 132, 136
OGTT. *See* Oral glucose tolerance
test
Olanzapine (Zyprexa), 137
Oral antidiabetic medication, 28–34,
29–30, 117–118
Oral glucose tolerance test (OGTT),
119
Oral insulin, 70
Overweight, 6–7, 8–9, 14

Pancreas, *4,* 34–35, 67, 124
Pancreatitis, *5*
Parents
of diabetic adolescents, 108–109
of diabetic children, 97–106
Partnership for Prescription
Assistance, 27, 93, 145
Patient. *See* Client
Patient Health Questionnaire
(PHQ-9), 133
Peer pressure, on prepubescent child
with diabetes, 104–105
Phases, for new diabetes medication,
72–74, *73*
PHQ-9. *See* Patient Health
Questionnaire
Physical activity, 15, 21–26, 122, 125,
139–140. *See also* Exercise
Physical limitations, on compliance
with diabetes management, 145
Pioglitazone (Actos), *30,* 32–34
Placebo effect, 72
Plans, for management of diabetes
in school-aged children,
100–104
Porcine insulin, 37
Positive reinforcement, for diabetes
education, 93
Pramlintide (Symlin), 44–45, *45*
Prandase. *See* Acarbose

Prandin. *See* Repaglinide
PRAR-gamma, 66–67
Precose. *See* Acarbose
Prediabetes, 1, *5,* 7–8, 12, 52–53
Prednisone, *5,* 7, 56, 80
Pregestational diabetes, 115–118
Pregnancy, diabetes during, *5,* 7, 36, 42, 56, 115–124
Prepubescent child, with diabetes, 104–106
Prescription assistance, 27–28, 93, 145
Prescriptions, costs of, 27–28, 93, 144–145
Prevalence
  of depression, 133
  of type 2 diabetes, 124
Prevention
  of autoimmune destruction, 65–67
  of type 1 diabetes, 65–70
  of type 2 diabetes, 12, 71–74
Problem solving, for diabetes care, 92
Procardia. *See* Nifedipine
Proinsulin, 67
Protamine, 37
Proteins, dietary, 12, 14, 17
Psychiatric disorder. *See* Mental illness
Puberty, diabetes during, 107
Pumping, of insulin, 35, 40, 42–44, 84–85, 126–127

Questionnaire
  for diabetes clients, *86–88*
  for diabetes mellitus client, *90–91*
  for mental health, 133
Questran. *See* Cholestyramine
Quetiapine (Seroquel), 137

Random blood glucose, 8
Rapid-acting insulin, *38*
Readiness to learn, of diabetes client, 88
Rebellion, against diabetes management, 105, 108, 109

Regeneration, of beta cells, 69–70
Rehabilitation Act of 1973, 102
Reinforcement. *See* Positive reinforcement
Religious constraints, on diabetes management, 149
Renal disease, 36, 126
Repaglinide (Prandin), 28–31, *29,* 31, 34, 57
Research, for new diabetes medications or products, 65–74
Resistance. *See* Insulin resistance
Responsibility, in adolescents with diabetes, 108–109
Retinopathy, *25*
Riomet. *See* Metformin
Risk factors
  for developing depression, 131–134
  for developing diabetes, 6–9, *15,* 119–120, 131–132, 137
Risperdal. *See* Risperidone
Risperidone (Risperdal), 137
Ritalin, 58
Rosiglitazone (Avandia), *30,* 32–34, 47, 66
Rosiglitazone/metformin (Avandamet), *30,* 32–33
Rule of 15, 84

Saturated fats, 13
Schizophrenia, diabetes and, 129, 135–137
School-aged child, diabetes in, 100–104
Screening
  for depression, 133–134
  for diabetes, 8–9, 119
Secretagogues, 28–31, 33, 57–58, *60*
Selective serotonin reuptake inhibitors (SSRIs), 135
Self-determination, of clients with diabetes, 154–156

Self-management
for adolescents with diabetes,
107–112
for children with diabetes, 97–106
for clients with mental illness,
139–140
of diabetes, 77–156
major components of, 80–81, *81*
self-determination in, 154–156
teaching of, 79–95, *89*
Sensors, for glucose, 61–62
Seroquel. *See* Quetiapine
Shoes, for exercise, 26
Short-acting insulin, *38*
Sick-day management, 18–19
Sirolimus, 68
Sneaking, in prepubescent children,
104–105
Special needs, diabetes in adults with,
115–127
SSRIs. *See* Selective serotonin
reuptake inhibitors
Stages, of grief, 150
*Standards of Medical Care in
Diabetes* (ADA), 12, 79
Starlix. *See* Nateglinide
Steroids, 68, 133
Stress, 54–56, 132
Strips, for blood glucose testing,
59–60, 125
Sugar, intake of, 13
Suicide, 153
Sulfonylureas, 28, *29,* 32, 34, 45, 58,
117
Supplies, for diabetes, 43, 59–60
Support system, for clients with
diabetes, 149–150
Survival skills, for diabetes clients, *81*
Symlin. *See* Pramlintide
Symptoms
of depression, 132–133
of diabetes, 8, 53, 97, 99
of hyperglycemia, *101*
of hypoglycemia, 56–57, *101*

of ketoacidosis, 53–54
of low literacy, 146–147
of mental illness, 135–136, 139
Syndrome X. *See* Metabolic
syndrome

Tacrolimus, 68
TCAs. *See* Tricyclic antidepressants
T cells, 66. *See also* Natural killer T
cells
Teachable moments, 85
Teacher
evaluation of, 93–95
nurse as, 79–95
*Teaching Nursing in an Associate
Degree Program,* 85
Teenagers, with diabetes, 107–112
Testing, of blood sugar, 18–19,
119–120. *See also* Monitoring
Therapeutic relationship, 89, 155
Thiazide diuretics, *5*
Thiazolidinediones, *30, 31–34*
Thyroxin, 56
Toddlers, with diabetes, 99–100
Tolerance, in autoimmune disorders,
66
Trans fatty acids, 13–14
Transplantation, as diabetes cure,
67–69
Treatment
for comorbid diabetes and
depression, 134–135
for low blood sugar, 57
medical nutritional therapy for,
11–19
medication for, 27–49
physical activity for, 21–26
Tricyclic antidepressants (TCAs),
135
Troglitazon (Rezulin), 33, 72, 74
Type 1.5 diabetes, 1
Type 1 diabetes, 1, *5,* 6, 9, 35, 40–41,
45, 47, 51–52, 58–60, 65–70, 107,
115–117, 122–124, 152

Type 2 diabetes, 1, *5*, 6–7, 9, 12, 28, 32–33, 35–36, 40–41, 45, 47–48, 51–52, 59–60, 71–74, 107, 117–118, 120–121, 123–124, 126–127, 136–137, 151–152, 154

Ultralente insulin (Humulin U), 37, *39*

Valproates (Depakote), 137
Volunteering, for clinical trials, 72–74

Waist circumference, *15*
Water, intake of, 25
Weight control, 22
Weight gain, 28, 32, 33, 48, 116, 135–137
Weight loss, 14–15, 44, 117

Ziprasidone (Geodon), 137
Zonulin inhibitor (AT-1001), 65
Zyprexa. *See* Olanzapine